Hypothyroidism - The Best Darn Complete Look

Two Popular Hypothyroid Resources Combined

By: James M. Lowrance   © 2013

SECTION ONE

A Complete Look
at Hypothyroidism

Underactive Thyroid Symptoms
and Treatments

TABLE OF CONTENTS:

INTRODUCTION:

Hypothyroidism is the medical term for an under-active thyroid gland. Hypothyroid disorders account for about 80% of thyroid disease cases, with the other 20% being hyperthyroid disorders (overactive thyroid). In this book, I will be addressing the subjects of symptoms, diagnosis and treatments for hypothyroidism. Within the chapters that follow, I will also be discussing blood tests and other diagnostic methods for detecting under-functioning thyroid glands and aspects of thyroid hormone replacement therapy. It is my hope that this e-book provides the reader with a general education on the subject of hypothyroidism.

CHAPTER ONE

Symptoms and Diagnosis of Hypothyroidism

Thyroid diseases affect an estimated 28,000,000 Americans and 80% of these have "hypothyroidism" or a low-functioning thyroid gland. According to medical experts, including the AACE (American Association of Clinical Endocrinologists) about half of those with thyroid hormone imbalances, remain undiagnosed. This is likely due to a combination of both lack of diagnostic testing being ordered by doctors and a lack of public education in regard to recognizing hypothyroid and hyperthyroid symptoms. Two major thyroid hormones, called T-3 (triiodothyronine) and T-4 (thyroxine), regulate the metabolism of every cell of our body. When the thyroid gland produces a lack of these, due to hindrance from a disease process it is experiencing or for any other reason, the body experiences "hypothyroidism", resulting in a slowed-down metabolism (reduced energy within all bodily cells).

Americans should become better educated in regard to the symptoms of hypothyroidism and the tests ordered for diagnosing it, so that they can recognize it and receive the needed treatment from a licensed physician.

One way in which public awareness is being gained, is via "Thyroid Awareness Month", which occurs each year, during the month of January. Medical groups and patient advocates use the month to place extra push behind spreading information to the general population in regard to recognizing thyroid disorders, which are more common than diabetes and heart disease combined.

Symptoms of Hypothyroidism

When a person is experiencing bodily-symptoms they may suspect hypothyroidism if one or more of them match the following, which are commonly listed for an under-active thyroid gland:

• Feeling cold in warm temperatures

• Dry skin and brittle fingernails

• Hair that becomes brittle and breaks off or falls out

• Thinning of the eyebrows and loss of the outer 1/3 portion of them

• Unexplained weight gain with no diet change

• Constipation

• Slowed heart rate and breathing

• Depression

• Physical tiredness/fatigue

• Feeling a fullness or tightness in the throat (a sign of goiter)

If you experience any of these symptoms, you should see your doctor and describe them to him/her, in-detail and ask if blood tests might be needed to diagnose or rule out the problem as being hypothyroidism, in addition to other tests that might be recommended. Other medical conditions can mimic hypothyroidism, including diabetes, nutritional deficiencies and sex hormone imbalances and so a qualified doctor can determine the testing that is needed. Even with this being the fact, patient-input regarding testing that may be needed, should be welcomed by doctors who want to see a reasonable degree of proactiveness from their patients and who see them as partners in their ongoing health care.

Tests for Hypothyroidism

While the symptoms and signs listed previously, point to possible thyroid disease and specifically to potential hypothyroidism, it is important once they are recognized as signs of a slowed metabolism, to have all of the proper blood tests ordered. Blood testing is the single most effective method, for detecting many common health disorders and diseases that exists in the field of professional medicine and this is certainly true of detecting thyroid dysfunction as well.

Thorough-evaluation thyroid testing comes in a grouping of tests called a "thyroid panel". These tests of thyroid hormone levels, include a test of the "TSH" level, which is a pituitary hormone ("Thyroid Stimulating Hormone" -- also called "thyrotropin") that the master endocrine brain-gland sends to the thyroid gland, stimulating it to produce the correct amount of thyroid hormones that are needed by the body to regulate metabolism. This is the reason it is called a "stimulating hormone" and when it becomes elevated above the normal range, this means the thyroid is falling behind in producing adequate hormones to supply the body. Some doctors actually use the TSH alone, in testing patients for hypothyroidism and also for an overactive thyroid (hyperthyroidism).

This is because of its sensitivity in detecting abnormal thyroid function earlier than any other thyroid function test. This pituitary hormone will sometimes detect hypothyroidism, even before the actual thyroid hormones do (before the T-3 and T-4 fall outside of normal limits).

Differences between Diagnostic and Treatment TSH

I have received a number of e-mails from thyroid patients responding to articles I have written over the years, which were on the subject of "TSH blood testing". They are complaining of not feeling well, in spite of being on thyroid medication and have included their most recent, follow-up lab results in their e-mails to me. In almost every one of these, their TSH levels are within the "normal" range for diagnosing hypothyroidism but they are not within the normal range for treating hypothyroidism and incredibly, they are stating that their Doctors are telling them that there is no difference between the two. There is a difference between the two however; and we only need to look at reliable medical sources to recognize this fact.

The "diagnostic" TSH levels, as revised and recommended by the AACE, in 2002 are roughly 0.3 to 3.0.

The "treatment" TSH level they recommend, is 1.0 to 2.0 for titrating hormone replacement therapy (adjusting thyroid medication levels in hypothyroid patients) however, many patients feel better, at the 1.0 and even down to the lowest TSH normal level of just above 0.3. Some patients even need a TSH that is slightly below the normal treatment level, due to slightly sluggish pituitary function that causes a TSH level that doesn't accurately represent the actual thyroid hormone levels but these cases require close monitoring by their Doctors. When the pituitary gland is actually under functioning, this is referred to as "hypopituitarism" however, some people may have subclinical forms of this problem that in some cases eventually causes a condition called "Central Hypothyroidism" (more on this subject in a succeeding chapter). For the general population of hypothyroid patients, the treatment range of 1.0 to 2.0 is the standard, among the top thyroid doctors .

Unfortunately, if a Doctor uses the diagnostic TSH range, a patient may be receiving inadequate treatment because this would mean that he or she would recognize even the highest-normal TSH, as being sufficient treatment, when it is most often not adequate for restoring a normal metabolism.

For example, if a patient is treated on thyroid hormone replacement medication and their treatment dose only suppresses their TSH down to 3.0, the Doctor who is not using the treatment TSH guideline but rather the diagnostic range, will recognize this level as being sufficient and the patient may continue to experience hypothyroid symptoms. This scenario is worsened, when the blood testing lab a Doctor is using, still abides by the old "diagnostic" TSH level of 0.5 to 5.0, revised by the AACE, in 2002 as previously mentioned, that helps diagnose developing hypothyroidism, being the current 0.3 to 3.0. Many labs have adjusted their ranges but some have set their high-normal cut-off value, somewhere between the old range and the revised one, such as having an upper-limit of "4.0". This is still considerable improvement over the former 5.0 and 6.0 values that most labs formerly adhered-to.

During my first two years of treatment for hypothyroidism, my first Doctor kept my TSH between 3.01 and 4.95 and stated that even that higher level was a "perfect reading". In reality, it was not only inadequate thyroid dosing, but I was virtually spinning-my-wheels and getting very little accomplished in reducing my hypothyroid symptoms.

Once finding a better-informed Doctor, who placed
me on combination T-4/T-3 replacement hormone
medication and dosing me, to reduce my TSH level to
between 0.5 and 1.0, I felt better than I had in my first
three years of treatment.

The Endocrinologist, who treats me currently, agrees
with other thyroid specialists who treat patients
optimally, by getting their TSH levels down to lowest
normal values. A thyroid patient forum I previously
posted at a great deal, that has a Board Certified
Endocrinologist answering questions on, repeatedly
confirmed that his patients felt better with a TSH
around 1.0 and that many of them he replaced with
doses that would suppress their TSH levels down to
between 0.5 and 1.0.

Thyroid Panels

A "thyroid panel" will also include a test of the actual
thyroid hormone levels, which are the "T-4," also
called the "thyroxine level", containing four iodine
molecules and the "T-3," also called the
"triiodothyronine level", containing three iodine
molecules. The T-4 is referred to in medical sources
as a "reserve hormone" and as a "precursor hormone".

While it helps the body with metabolism at the tissue-level, it also converts into the more active T-3 hormone, which is several times more powerful than the T-4 hormone (by 5 to 10 times) and is more active in regulating the body's metabolism. Either one of these two hormones or a combination of the two being found low in the blood, indicates hypothyroidism. If the TSH is also high, with either of these being low, this, too, indicates hypothyroidism. Even if these two thyroid hormones are in the normal range but TSH is elevated, this too can indicate hypothyroidism.

The T-4 and T-3 blood tests come in a variety of different versions, such as the "totals" of each, the "free" levels of each or may be combined in tests called the "FTI Index" or the "T-7". There is also one called the "T-3 Uptake". All of these help to determine thyroid hormone production levels and all of them have lab ranges with a "below-normal" indicating hypothyroidism and an "above-normal" indicating hyperthyroidism.

A 24 hour Thyroid Uptake Scan is another test of thyroid function that doctors sometimes use to detect hypothyroidism (more frequent used for diagnosing hyperthyroid disorders).

The patient being tested will receive a dose of radioactive iodine, administered by a doctor or a lab technician, that is absorbed by the thyroid gland. The radiological imaging that follows reveals how well the thyroid is functioning, by highlighting the tissues within the gland. It does this by revealing how well iodine is absorbed by the gland and whether this is occurring evenly or if part of the gland is failing. An Uptake Scan can determine how well the thyroid functions to a highly accurate estimated percentage-level.

CHAPTER TWO

Common Causes of Hypothyroidism

When it is determined that a patient has hypothyroidism, the doctor will then further investigate to find the cause of the low functioning thyroid gland. The most common cause found in patients with hypothyroidism in the industrialized countries of the world, is an immune system response that is referred to as "thyroid autoimmunity". "Hashimoto's thyroiditis" is the usual term applied to this cause although, there are other variations, such as "Ord's thyroiditis" (the latter being a more common finding in countries of the UK). The condition is also medically known as "chronic lymphocytic thyroiditis" and results in a slow destruction of the gland, rendering it unable to provide the body with ample amounts of thyroid hormones. Some Hashimoto's patients also experience goiters but they are usually mild, while those with Ord's actually see their thyroid glands shrink (atrophy) over time.

Hashimoto's Thyroiditis

The majority of patients with both hypothyroidism (under-active thyroid) and hyperthyroidism (overactive thyroid) are experiencing autoimmune diseases that cause these conditions.

Hypothyroidism-The Best Darn Complete Look

16

When the autoimmune disease of the thyroid causes hyperthyroidism, it is called "Grave's Disease". I discuss the symptoms, causes, diagnosis and treatments for hyperthyroid conditions, in the book titled *"A Complete Look at Hyperthyroidism"*.

The immune system normally sends out antibodies, which are killer cells designed to eradicate foreign invaders from the body that can make us sick. These invaders include viruses, bacteria and allergens. The purpose of antibodies is to seek these out and to destroy them, to prevent our bodies from becoming ill. The problem with "thyroid antibodies" is that, like other antibodies that cause autoimmune diseases, they are eventually directed against normal tissues such as the thyroid gland as if it is one of these invaders. It is a case of mistaken identity that over time causes damage to the thyroid gland via ongoing cell death. Eventually, the antibodies will actually kill-out the thyroid gland completely over time, turning its healthy tissue into an unhealthy type that no longer absorbs iodine from the diet, in order to manufacture its metabolism-regulating hormones.

As previously-mentioned, thyroid autoimmunity means your gland is being attacked by antibodies that are sent from the immune system that have the goal of destroying it.

This autoimmune process not only damages the thyroid gland but it also causes inflammation within it, which is where the "thyroiditis" term comes from. The antibodies can also serve to block some of the thyroid hormone produced by the gland, so that it doesn't do the job it needs to, even when there is near-ample levels available in the body. Patients can have varying symptoms at the early stage of autoimmune hypothyroidism, such as the subclinical types (not full blown) and the overt types (full blown). As mentioned earlier, it is the most common cause of a low functioning thyroid in many industrialized countries of the world, including the US, second only to iodine deficiency hypothyroidism which is more prominent in less-developed countries that all-combined, represent a majority of the world-population.

Diagnosis of Hashimoto's Thyroiditis

Patients suspected of having this autoimmune form of thyroid disease, need to be tested for thyroid antibodies, in addition to being tested for low levels of thyroid hormone. In some cases, these antibody tests can reveal that autoimmune thyroid disease is going on, in patients with normal range thyroid hormone levels.

The tests that help detect Hashimoto's thyroiditis, are the "anti-TPO" (anti-thyroidperoxidase) and the "anti-TG" (anti-thyroglobulin) and sometimes also the "TSI" antibodies (thyroid stimulating immunoglogulin), although these latter mentioned ones are more commonly found positive in patients with Graves' disease. People with developing autoimmune hypothyroidism (Hashimoto's thyroiditis), can have elevated antibody levels that cause them a degree of symptoms, even when thyroid hormones levels fall within normal-range.

Medical research articles by reputable medical groups, state this fact regarding the disease process itself, involving thyroid antibodies as being a factor in causing symptoms in Hashimoto's patients. These research articles conclude that elevated levels of these immune cells can cause fibromyalgia and other rheumatic types of symptoms in persons with only sub-clinical hypothyroidism. Some of these articles also state that autoimmune thyroid disease can have a degree of systemic (system-wide) effect, so that the immune system response affects not only the thyroid gland area but other parts of the body as well.

Following is a quote from an article published on the PubMed website (U.S. National Institutes of Health).

The article states that the autoimmunity aspect of the disease, rather than abnormal thyroid hormone levels alone, are what contribute to the symptoms of Hasihimoto's disease:

"A variety of rheumatic manifestations have been described in association with autoimmune thyroiditis. In the past, most of these manifestations were attributed to the underlying thyroid dysfunction, in particular hypothyroidism. However, a responsibility of the mechanisms involved in the autoimmunity rather than a direct action of thyroid hormones seems supported by the evidences that some rheumatic manifestations may occur even in euthyroid patients, or that they are more frequent in hypothyroid patient with autoimmune thyroiditis than in those without this disease.

Rheumatic manifestations could be sometimes attributable to the autoimmune rheumatic diseases frequently associated with autoimmune thyroiditis, such as Sjögren's syndrome, rheumatoid arthritis, systemic lupus erythematosus, or scleroderma. Among the most important or frequent rheumatic manifestations there are a mild non-erosive variety of arthritis, polyarthralgia, myalgia, and sicca syndrome without a true Sjögren's syndrome.

Although the possible pathogenesis of these manifestations is not completely established, some hypotheses may be proposed, including a role of autoantibodies characteristics of autoimmune thyroiditis, a possible overlap between autoimmune thyroiditis and some autoimmune rheumatic diseases, and a systemic inflammatory reaction associated with thyroiditis."

(From the research article titled: "Chronic autoimmune thyroiditis and rheumatic manifestations." - Online Link Location: http://www.ncbi.nlm.nih.gov/pubmed/15288851)

Hashitoxicosis

Patients with Hashimoto's thyroiditis can also go through phases of temporary hyperthyroidism, before the onset of progressive hypothyroidism sets in and the term for this related condition is "Hashitoxicosis". These patients are the ones mentioned previously, who might need to be blood tested for TSI antibodies because the hyperthyroid phases they go through are due to having some elevation of these antibodies, that normally cause Grave's Disease (autoimmune hyperthyroidism), in addition to the ones that cause Hashimoto's thyroiditis (Anti-TPO and Anti-TG).

Here is a quote from an online resource in regard to Hashitoxicosis:

"Hashitoxicosis is an autoimmune thyroid disorder, in which individuals with autoimmune hypothyrodism, usually Hashimoto's thyroiditis (HT), experience intermittent or sporadic periods where they also have symptoms of hyperthyrodism." (Grave's Disease and Hyperthyroidism Wiki)

You could almost say that these patients are suffering from Grave's and Hashimoto's, simultaneously. Even without having the TSI antibodies present, Hashimoto's patients can experience flares of thyroiditis (spells of increased thyroid inflammation), which can also cause mild hyperthyroid type symptoms that are not as severe as those caused by Hashitoxicosis but that are still concerning. Not all medical sources agree on this aspect and some believe that Hashitoxicosis can only be identified as such if hyperthyroid symptoms are severe, rather than mild, as can be the case with episodes of thyroiditis.

Central Hypothyroidism

Hypothyroidism can also be caused by a failure in the chain of communication between the glands that work in-sync with each other.

These glands normally result in the proper release of thyroid hormone from the thyroid gland. The "pituitary gland", a major brain-gland actually sends messages to the thyroid gland using the messenger hormone called "TSH". If there is a problem within the pituitary gland in being able to stimulate the thyroid, such as an obstructive tumor that develops within it, causing it to also be low functioning (hypopituitarism), the cause would then be referred to as "Central Hypothyroidism".

Other Secondary Causes

In more complicated cases, hypothyroidism might be secondary to another disease process in the body, in which case, extensive blood testing of all types may need to be undertaken to determine the underlying cause of the thyroid hormone imbalance or what is also referred to as "Secondary Hypothyroidism".

Certain types of illnesses and severe, chronic stress, can cause the body to convert too much of the T-4 hormone into an inactive form of hormone called "Reverse T-3" (T-4 normally converts into adequate amounts of the active T-3), which will cause a person to experience a type of "hypothyroidism", due to low T-3 hormone in the body.

This type of hypothyroidism that is secondary to an illness or from severe stress in the body is also referred to as "Sick Euthyroid Syndrome" or "low T-3 Syndrome" and is also sometimes referred to as "Wilson's Temperature Syndrome". It is usually a temporary form of hypothyroidism that can be corrected with short term T-3 hormone replacement therapy. This type of hypothyroidism is rare compared to the types that are caused by a diseased thyroid gland or "primary hypothyroidism".

Postpartum Hypothyroidism

When women experience low thyroid hormone after pregnancy, following giving birth, the term for this type of under-active thyroid is "postpartum hypothyroidism". This type happens in about 10% of new mothers within 12 months of giving birth and for some it improves on its own, without treatment. Others may require short-term treatment with thyroid hormone replacement. If the hypothyroidism that is triggered by pregnancy is the autoimmune type, the treatment for it will likely be life-long and the pregnancy simply brought the disease to the surface, which would have eventually manifested on its own over time.

24

Iodine Deficiency Hypothyroidism

One common acquired type of hypothyroidism that occurs in countries where diets are low in iodine is referred to as "iodine deficiency hypothyroidism". This type is rare in industrialized countries, so is more common in those considered to be "third world countries" (less developed and less industrialized and usually poverty level).

You don't often hear of people getting their iodine levels checked because iodine doesn't necessarily tell you anything about your thyroid function. The iodine level in the body can fluctuate considerably, due to what is in your diet (i.e. consuming high iodine foods like kelp etc...) or because of supplements you take that contain iodine. The real tests of thyroid function are the actual thyroid hormone levels; T-4 and T-3 (preferably the "free levels") and the TSH level which is the pituitary hormone previously discussed, that is highly sensitive in monitoring thyroid function via blood testing.

In regard to high iodine content foods or supplements containing iodine, I suggest not consuming these for several days before being evaluated for thyroid function via blood testing because iodine can work adversely in some people with autoimmune thyroid disease.

It can cause fluctuations in thyroid antibodies and hormone levels, giving a false impression of how a patients thyroid function is actually running. Iodine is the treatment for hypothyroidism caused by iodine deficiency but this type is almost non-existent in industrialized countries that manufacture iodized table salt. While there is some disagreement regarding this fact, it is believed that use of iodized salt alone usually contains as much iodine as average, healthy people need for proper thyroid function.

Following Thyroid Removal

Hyperthyroid patients, who have their thyroid glands either surgically removed (thyroidectomy) or destroyed by a process called "Radioactive Iodine Ablation", to halt their hyperthyroidism, will afterward become hypothyroid, with their glands no longer being present to manufacture thyroid hormones. They will afterward have to be given thyroid hormone replacement therapy just as patients who become hypothyroid due to any of the other previously listed reasons.

CHAPTER THREE

Treatment for Hypothyroidism

The treatment for hypothyroidism is simply to
"replace" the low hormone levels and to restore what
is needed by the body to regain a normal metabolism
(rate at which the body uses energy from food, water
and oxygen). This is done by giving the patient
"thyroid hormone replacement medication". The
Doctor will prescribe a starting dose for the patient
and do follow-up blood re-testing to adjust the dose to
the correct level over time, which is called "titrating"
the dose -- the goal being to reach the most optimized
levels possible.

Most patients with hypothyroidism are prescribed a T-
4 only brand of thyroid hormone medication (e.i.
Synthroid and brands of Levothyroxine) and the also
needed T-3 hormone is converted from it, within the
body successfully. In patients with a less-common
problem called "impaired conversion" however, a T-4
only hormone medication will not supply them with
adequate T-3 that is also needed in the body. If this
problem exists, it will be evident by their blood test
results that monitor their dose.

If a patient's T-4 to T-3 ratio is off too much they may need a thyroid hormone replacement medication that contains both T-4 and T-3 hormones (e.i. Armour Thyroid or Thyrolar) or they may need the addition of a T-3 medication (e.i. Cytomel) to the T-4 only brand they are already taking. There are also people who by taking a T-4/T-3 combination drug, elevate their Free T-3 level too high and have to be switched to a T-4 only medication. This is why it is important for hypothyroid patients to be treated by qualified doctors, who can determine the type of thyroid hormone medication that is best-suited for them.

Armour Thyroid Vs Other Natural Hypothyroidism Treatments

"Armour Thyroid" brand of prescribed hypothyroid therapy medication has a set dose of hormone, just like synthetic does. It contains 38mcg of T-4 (levothyroxin) 9mcg of T-3 (liothyronine) per each grain (60mg tablet). The only change the medication makes once it enters the body is that the T-4 in it, will partially convert into more T-3, if the body determines it needs more. The other change would be the percent of absorption of it that can be affected by other things a patient is consuming at the time of taking their dose.

Taking calcium or iron for example, within 6-hours of taking thyroid medication (either type), can limit its absorption in the body, as can too much dietary fiber, so these need to be consumed about 6 hours apart from taking the daily thyroid hormone dose.

There has been ongoing misinformation being published, in regard to the Armour brand not being consistent in doses however, Forest Pharmaceuticals, the manufacturer, has been cleared by the FDA for not having dosage inconsistencies within their tablets. Synthroid recently had to go through the same scrutiny and approval regarding pill-dose accuracy and so these accusations regarding dose-inconsistencies that sometime arise are likely fueled by pharmaceutical wars for market shares, more than anything else. The Forest Company, who makes Armour, also makes synthetic T-4, just like Knoll Pharmaceuticals, the maker of Synthroid does. They also make a combo synthetic T-4 & T-3 combo (Thyrolar).

I am not recommending Armour over Synthroid because I believe some patients do better on Synthroid, however, I also believe Armour is given an undeserved "bad rap", by Doctors who are simply parroting what the Pharmaceutical companies are telling them.

The fact is that Synthroid has had bad press on it at times, just as Armour has. I maintain my own belief that patients need trial-regimens of the opposite type medication, if they are tried on one and are not having success with it, via adequate or optimal symptom relief.

Prescribed thyroid hormones take-over for the thyroid gland, so that it atrophies (stops working) and this is actually the whole point of thyroid hormone replacement therapy. If a person waits until the thyroid gland completely stops functioning before starting thyroid medication, they risk serious health issues or even death by myxedema coma. This is the dilemma, even for Doctors, in knowing at what point to actually start mildly-hypothyroid patients on hormone replacement because it always results in the eventual shut down of their own thyroid glands.

Symptoms are one of the most important reasons medication needs to be started but also, to help reduce elevated thyroid antibody levels (this sometimes takes years to achieve optimally) and to prevent goiter (swelling) and nodules (tumor-like growths) from developing within the gland and so we can see that there are multiple reasons for starting medication in patients with developing hypothyroidism.

Many medical resources state that thyroid medications help to reduce antibodies over time (opposite of what others claim – that it can increase them). If antibody levels increase despite being on medication, this does not necessarily mean the medication is the cause of this but it could also be due to thyroiditis flares that happen commonly with autoimmune hypothyroid disease. The point to all this being that it is unavoidable to take hormone replacement medication if you have Hashimoto's disease as the cause of hypothyroidism because it is very rarely ever reversed and it is usually progressive.

Thyroid Boosters versus Hormone Replacement

There are companies who market non-prescription natural "thyroid supplements" and they know many Doctors will not approve these in combination with thyroid hormone replacement and so they claim these should be taken <u>instead</u> of a medically prescribed drug. It's very possible that these help to boost thyroid function for a while but to claim they will reverse autoimmune thyroid disease is false. If there were supplements that could do this, medical research would have discovered it many years ago.

While I believe there are natural supplements that can definitely improve a person's thyroid function, I do not believe they can replace thyroid hormone replacement medications, needed by patients with advanced disease of the gland that has already caused moderate or overt hypothyroidism. It is my opinion, and one I know also agrees with that of most medical professionals, that trying to replace thyroid hormone medication, containing actual thyroid hormone with a supplement containing no thyroid hormone, or an inconsistent amount, could actually be dangerous. Lack of thyroid hormone in the body, must be replaced and a patient cannot depend upon a supplement instead, that is supposed to increase thyroid function when the thyroid has lost ground that cannot be regained, once it is permanently damaged due to a disease process.

One has to be careful to read the ingredients of supplements being considered because Endocrinologists often warn patients that these "thyroid supplements" that contain no hormone, will not treat hypothyroidism and some contain ingredients that may actually work adversely with thyroid medications, including iodine. The fact is that autoimmune thyroid disease cannot be reversed except in very rare cases.

This would mean that even if those supplements worked to help strengthen the thyroid gland, how long would this improvement last? If the thyroid starts going downhill again once these supplements were stopped, this would mean they would have to be lifelong treatment as well. If antibodies continued to attack the thyroid while one is on these non-hormone supplements, the gland would still eventually become so damaged over time, that there is no way they could continue to restore its function.

Best TSH Treatment Level

As briefly mentioned previously, the AACE (Endocrine Society/Thyroid Specialists) and other medical authorities recommend that hypothyroid patient's TSH levels while on thyroid hormone replacement medication, be suppressed down to between "1.0 and 2.0". The TSH level rises, when thyroid hormone decreases and it falls when the thyroid hormone levels increase. If a patient's TSH is not kept below 2.0, they risk continued hypothyroid symptoms (patients can vary in their needs) and if it is brought significantly below 1.0, they risk patients developing hyperthyroid symptoms (dose-induced thyrotoxicity).

33

Some Endocrinologists actually keep some patient's TSH levels between, "0.3 to 1.0" (lowest normal) if they feel the patient has a slightly sluggish pituitary gland or is simply a patient who does not fit into the general population in regard to their TSH level. These type cases, take careful monitoring by treating doctors as also previously mentioned.

CHAPTER FOUR

The Pros and Cons of Hypothyroid Treatment

Patients, who are diagnosed with hypothyroidism and are being treated for it with hormone replacement therapy, can sometimes have other imbalances that hinder the effectiveness of their treatment. Things such as adrenal hormones being low or low levels of ferritin/iron, Vitamin B-12 etc... (elements needed for strong blood), can cause thyroid hormone treatment, to be less effective in patients with imbalances of these and this is why thorough blood testing of all major nutritional levels may need to be done, to find any problems that prevent the treatment from working as well.

Tips for Taking Thyroid Hormone Medication for Best Results

People taking thyroid hormone replacement medication for hypothyroidism need to follow a set-routine for taking their daily dose. Hormone therapy can have a delicate balance and even small variations in the levels within the body can greatly affect how well a patient feels.

The steps described following, help to insure the best results from thyroid hormone replacement therapy.

Take your thyroid hormone medication on an empty stomach, with plenty of water. Many patients find it easier to take their thyroid medication on an empty stomach by doing so first thing in the morning before having breakfast. Once the medication has been taken, it is recommended that a patient wait at least 30 minutes before eating, to allow the medication time to be absorbed adequately within the digestive tract. Taking the medication with a full glass of water also helps with digestion and absorption of the medication.

Take your thyroid hormone medication at the same time each day. When you take your thyroid medication at the same time each day, this helps your hormone levels remain more stable than if you take it at different times each day. Most thyroid medications have a long half-life of several days (those containing T3 have a half-life of only a few hours). Even very small changes in the rhythm of your dosage can affect the way you feel. According to the manufacturers of thyroid medications, the hormone will peak in the body at a certain time after ingesting it and then remain stable for a period of time and afterward have a slightly lowered effect.

A patient will want to see the peak and stable effects during the day and the lowered effect toward the end of the day, as time for rest and sleep arrives after daily of activities.

If you take vitamins or supplements containing iron or calcium, be sure to take them six hours apart from your thyroid medication dose. As previously-mentioned, these two supplements can have a negative effect on thyroid hormone medication, by preventing it from fully absorbing in the body, if they are taken at the same time or too-close to the time of the hormone replacement dose. To prevent malabsorption, it is recommended that you take these supplements at least six hours apart from your thyroid medication each day (some sources suggest eight hours as added precaution). Some patients take their thyroid medication in the morning on an empty stomach and will take their supplements containing iron and/or calcium after lunch, six hours later, to prevent this problem.

When you have blood retests of your thyroid hormone levels, take your medication at the same time, to correlate with each blood draw. Some patients on the day of a blood draw (to retest their thyroid hormone levels) will skip their thyroid medication dose until after their blood is drawn.

Other patients will take their thyroid medication dose before the blood draw but will make sure the blood is drawn at the same time for each retest, to make sure levels are consistent in correlation with it. It really is not that important which method one may use, as long as they do-so consistently for each blood draw to retest their thyroid hormone levels while being treated for hypothyroidism.

Never adjust your own thyroid medication dose. There can be times when hypothyroid symptoms may manifest themselves despite the fact that you are taking your thyroid medication properly. This might make some patients believe that a slight increase in their dose that day would help to relieve these symptoms, and consequently they are tempted to take it upon themselves to increase their dose. This is never a good idea, without the consent and supervision of a doctor. Even small adjustments in a prescribed dose can alter hormone levels in the body, for days at a time. If a patient seems to be experiencing symptoms of low thyroid hormone or those of an overactive thyroid (too much hormone), they should report these to their doctor for instructions on adjusting their medication or in making an office visit for further evaluation of their treatment.

Hypothyroid Hormone Therapy Always Perfect?

I receive e-mails often from treated hypothyroid patients, in fact one I received from a woman recently who had not yet been started on treatment, stating that she repeatedly went to Doctors with the full array of hypothyroid symptoms and all of her thyroid hormone levels, including TSH were all within the normal range, even with repeated testing. She finally demanded antibody tests and her Doctor said that the results of these "were off the map", meaning they were very highly elevated, so he went ahead and placed her on thyroid medication because of her symptoms.

Many medical information sources state that Hashimoto's thyroiditis does not cause symptoms, only the resulting hypothyroidism, once detectable by abnormal thyroid hormone blood tests will cause symptoms. In my experience in corresponding with many hypothyroid patients by email and as a thyroid disease forum moderator, I have found that far too many untreated patients report symptoms before hormone levels fall outside the normal range, for this to be an uncommon experience. This also means that the same disease that results in already-treated patient's hypothyroidism can potentially continue to cause a degree of symptoms.

This may be true, even when hormone levels are corrected back into the normal range, even at optimal levels.

The description of expected results from thyroid medications, from those who state that thyroid autoimmunity is not a factor in symptoms, describe it in almost miraculous or magical terms such as one I read recently that stated to the effect; "once on thyroid hormone medication, any symptoms a patient has will resolve and the patient will return to normal within a few weeks". Improvement, yes! Symptoms completely resolved and a return to normal, not in all cases! A large percent of patients may see near-perfect results but for many, there is ongoing struggle with a degree of symptoms because autoimmune thyroiditis is a disease and is not cured by correcting the hypothyroidism that results from it, in fact no cure has yet been discovered.

We are thankful and grateful for the results we do experience from hormone replacement therapy but many in the medical community, need to be realistic with patients who can feel let down by anything less than what they are told will happen. If perfect-relief is not experienced, the patient is told "it is not their thyroid" and usually they will then be diagnosed with psychosomatic or emotional problems.

Emotions may very well be some of the symptoms that do not resolve completely with hypothyroid treatment. It is only fair to the patient however, for the emotional diagnosis to be described as being "thyroid related" if the symptoms manifested with their thyroid disease and the patient had no prior problems with them before the disease-onset. This may also be opportunity for the doctor to give the patient a trial of a different prescribed hormone, to see if it has better success with relieving their unresolved emotional symptoms.

I have also read some articles recently stating to the effect that "patients who do not see their symptoms resolve once optimized on thyroid hormone medication, are simply experiencing added stress and worry from the reality of having the disease". These are the type things that have given me a passion for this particular aspect of misinformation. It's hard to sit-still while literally thousands of thyroid patients are pegged with these unfair descriptions that simply are not true in most cases.

You would think from some of these descriptions, that this disease is just a mild condition similar to a cold, that is easily treatable and that seldom ever causes ongoing problems once treated.

41

This is why research articles about "the role of thyroid autoimmunity" in symptoms both physical and emotional and the "Health Related Quality of Life of Thyroid Patients" surveys that are being conducted are so important in my opinion.

Too many medical sources and thyroid medication manufacturers, still state simply that once a patient with Hashimoto's-hypothyroidism for example, is on replacement hormone, they will get better and no longer suffer symptoms, after about 6-weeks or so on a dose of the hormone medication. The fact is however, that many patients need several dose adjustments before reaching the proper level of replacement that restores them to a eutyhroid (normalized) state. This can take a process of many months as determined by each individual case and treating doctors should inform patients of this possibility. Patients should also be informed of the fact that "thyroid autoimmunity" has potential to contribute to symptoms in some patients, apart from corrected thyroid hormone levels.

While most patients do see significant improvement, many still suffer a degree of symptoms, no matter how optimized their treatment is because the medication does not cure the underlying autoimmune disease that causes the thyroid imbalance.

For this reason, patients should not be patronized and made to feel ridiculous or have it implied to them that they are hypochondriacs or experiencing psychosomatic symptoms, simply because they do not see complete relief of symptoms from thyroid replacement hormone therapy.

CHAPTER FIVE

My Personal Experience with Hypothyroidism

My story started at age 40, in early 2003, when I crashed into severe symptoms of thyroid disease and had no idea what it was. Mine followed a severe period of stress, which according to many patient-testimonials and medical research articles, can be a trigger for underlying thyroid disease to surface.

I visited a doctor who was filling-in for my regular doctor and she immediately diagnosed me with Generalized Anxiety Disorder and prescribed me an antidepressant, an anti-anxiety medication and a beta-blocker to control my adrenaline surges. My symptoms were: fatigue, post exertion malaise, brain fog, very dry skin, anxiety, depression, severe sweating, weight loss (rapid and temporary), joint aches and my hair was starting to break off and fall out in small amounts. The symptoms scared me out of my wits! I knew beyond a doubt that there were more than emotions going on in my body, so I demanded a blood draw and asked for my thyroid hormones, glucose and blood counts to be tested. I had the blood drawn before I started the antidepressant that was prescribed.

The Hospital lost my lab results for over a month and didn't bother to tell me and when I called about them after waiting to hear about my results through my Doctor's office, they said everything looked great and not to worry about it.

My own doctor, who was gone at the time I made the visit the fill-in doctor, returned for a short period of time before leaving again to become a missionary doctor in a foreign country. Just before he left, he was able to locate my lab results and wrote me a review letter in regard to them. His first sentence stated: "Your lab tests indicate you are low on thyroid hormone". He also pointed out that I was borderline diabetic. The hospital staff, who said my tests were normal, made me realize that you cannot take the word of someone other than a doctor in regard to medical issues and you need to see all of your own lab results (request copies – because you are entitled to them by law).

My TSH on the lab results, was elevated at "8.3" (lab range - 0.4 to 4.5) and my T-3 Uptake was several points below normal. I followed up with tests that revealed my hypothyroidism to be caused by Hashimoto's thyroiditis. My TG antibodies were at "537" (normal range <40) and my TPO antibodies were "120" (normal range <35).

I also found through other lab testing that my cortisol levels were low (adrenal fatigue) but an ACTH Stimulation test ruled out true (full blown) adrenal insufficiency.

I was started on Synthroid (synthetic T4) in 2003 and later switched to Armour Thyroid (natural T4 and T3) in 2004. My doctor who switched me thought I might be one of the rare cases of "inadequate T-4 to T-3 conversion" (a condition I mention briefly in a previous chapter) but actually I was under-dosed on the Synthroid. Regardless, I do well on Armour and now take 2.5 grains (150mg). I also take vitamins and supplements that help the adrenal fatigue that flares when I'm physically overactive or experiencing high stressor levels and/or prolonged stress.

I was also diagnosed with Non-alcoholic Fatty Liver Disease, caused by Metabolic Syndrome (an insulin resistance type condition). I continue to work on weight loss/control and improved diet, to avoid diabetes or worsening of the fatty liver. An important aspect of my treatment for all of my conditions is lifestyle changes (i.e. healthy diet, exercise, stress control and healthy supplements approved by my doctor).

My Experience with Hypothyroid Related Emotions

As I began developing hypothyroidism from autoimmune thyroid disease (Hashimoto's), I began having severe anxiety and panic attacks. Many patients experience these, just as the thyroid gland begins to fail and become hypothyroid (depression is also common). With Grave's Disease patients (Autoimmune-Hyperthyroidism), they-too will have the anxiety symptoms but many times these are continuous, until they can begin treatment to slow-down the overproduction of hormone by their thyroid glands.

My anxiety was intermittent and would alternate with spells of depression. Researchers describe anxiety symptoms from autoimmune hypothyroidism, as sometimes being caused by the gland's attempt to "sputter back to life" as it begins to fail in attempt to fight off the autoimmune attack. The actual medical term for this is "Hashitoxicosis" (short-term phases of hyperthyroidism) and patients will have it to varying degrees but it usually manifests in a milder form that can still cause significant anxiety symptoms. Milder flares might be better-termed as "thyroiditis flares" because true Hashitoxicosis would cause significant, long-term hyperthyroidism.

Following is a quote from Richard C. W. Hall, M.D., who points out the fact that anxiety is a common symptom found in newly diagnosed hypothyroid patients:

"The development of severe anxiety disorders in hypothyroid states are as much or more related to the rapidity of change of thyroid hormone levels as they are to the absolute levels encountered. Whether the cause of hypothyroidism is auto-immune or follows thyroidectomy, oblation of the gland by radioactive iodine, the ingestion of medicines such as lithium carbonate, or is associated with thyroid cancer, the neuropsychiatric symptoms are similar."

(From the Research Article Titled: "ANXIETY AND ENDOCRINE DISEASE" - Online Link Location: http://www.drrichardhall.com/anxiety.htm)

Symptoms of Anxiety

What are the symptoms of anxiety that can be experienced by thyroid patients? Following are some of the more common symptoms of anxiety in-general.

• sudden intense feelings of fear

• rapid heart rate

• elevated blood pressure

• rapid breathing (hyperventilation)

• sweating

• trembling

• muscle tension with pain (including chest area)

There can also be anxiety that is more of a constant type keyed-up feeling, called "free floating anxiety" that causes a continuous nervous feeling and one of being on-edge that thyroid patients can experience. This also brings on feelings of constant, chronic worry that is referred to as "Generalized Anxiety Disorder". The more intense episodes of anxiety come under the heading of "anxiety attacks" and "panic attacks". These obviously are very unpleasant and there were times I would experience these with my Hashimoto's disease, especially during the night, causing me to awaken in a cold sweat, while I also experienced other hyperthyroid type symptoms, including teporary weight loss from short-term Hashitoxicosis.

Symptoms of Depression

There are symptoms of depression that are common to thyroid disease patients as well, especially prior to being treated. The more common symptoms are:

• feeling slowed down

• inability to enjoy things

• sadness

• irritability

• anger

• feelings of hopelessness (sometimes including suicidal thoughts)

• feeling tired and lethargic

The symptoms of depression can co-exist with anxiety or sometimes will alternate so that a thyroid patient experiences anxiety part of the time and depression part of the time.

My emotional symptoms were some of the first to resolve with thyroid hormone replacement therapy.

I still have occasional mild to moderate flares of anxiety and depression symptoms due to having the autoimmune thyroid disease but the improvements over my pre-treatment state have been significant.

Thyroid patients suffering emotional symptoms should be encouraged to know that hormone replacement therapy can potentially improve these symptoms significantly. If it does not do-so adequately in some patients, there are additional medication-options out there that are effective in treating emotional symptoms as well (i.e. antidepressant and anti-anxiety drugs). Psychiatric therapies can also be helpful, such as "Cognitive Behavioral Therapy" and can be combined with drug therapies or administered as stand-alone treatments, depending on the needs of individual hypothyroid patients.

If you suspect that you might have hypothyroidism or hyperthyroidism, it is important that you see a qualified medical doctor for further evaluation. As is the case with most health disorders and diseases, treatments can be more effective and can prevent further complications, the sooner a diagnosis is made and treatment is started.

(END – SECTION ONE)

SECTION TWO

The Best Darn
Hypothyroidism Book!

Studies on the Underactive
Thyroid Gland

TABLE OF CONTENTS:

INTRODUCTION:

Covering the subject of hypothyroidism – an under active thyroid gland, this section contains 17 chapters dedicated to the most common thyroid disorder that exists. All aspects regarding hypothyroid conditions are addressed in this resource, in easy-to-understand language and is very possibly the best that is currently available on the subject.

CHAPTER ONE

Hypothyroidism Basic Facts

Underactive Thyroid Gland General Information

The American Association of Clinical Endocrinologists (AACE) estimates that approximately 27-million Americans suffer thyroid diseases and up to 13-million cases remain undiagnosed. Hypothyroid conditions account for about 80% of abnormal thyroid function cases. There are varied symptoms, causes, diagnostic methods and treatments for hypothyroidism.

When a person experiences hypothyroidism, meaning his or her thyroid hormone production has decreased to abnormally low levels (low T3 and/or T4) this results in the metabolism becoming slowed down. The resulting effects are signs and symptoms affecting every area of the body with the severity of them depending on how advanced the hypothyroidism is.

Major Causes of Hypothyroidism

Hypothyroidism can have causes that are "primary" (in the gland) or "secondary" (indirectly affecting the gland). The number one cause of hypothyroidism, worldwide is iodine deficiency which is due to the fact that third world countries (less industrialized) account for most of the world population.

These are areas where iodine is lacking in their diets. The thyroid gland depends on iodine for production of thyroid hormones. Part of this lack comes from their not having iodized salt as we do, who live in the more advanced countries of the world where iodized salt is more easily attainable.

Industrialized countries have "thyroid autoimmunity" as the most common cause of hypothyroidism. This would also be referred to as "chronic autoimmune thyroiditis", with most cases falling under the "Hashimoto's thyroiditis" umbrella.

Thyroid removal surgeries or procedures, in which part of the thyroid gland is removed as treatment for hyperthyroidism (overactive) or to remove thyroid nodules or large goiters, can also result in the need following, to replace thyroid hormone levels that become low afterward.

Other less-common causes of hypothyroidism include pregnancies and problems involving the major glands in the brain that regulate hormone production in the thyroid gland. These are the "hypothalamus" (sends TRH to the pituitary gland) and the "pituitary" (sends TSH to the thyroid, in response to TRH). These glands work in a continuous loop unless disrupted by tumors that can develop within them with hypothyroidism being the end result when the process is hindered, also called "Central Hypothyroidism".

Hypothyroid Symptoms

A slowed metabolism from hypothyroidism can cause an array of symptoms. These include:

• joint and muscle aches

• depression

• fatigue and low energy

• dry skin

• hair loss

• constipation

• weight gain

• water retention

• swelling in the body (edema)

• slowed heart rate and breathing

• heavier menstrual cycles

• elevated cholesterol

• goiter and changes in appetite

Symptom severity varies depending on the progression of hypothyroidism.

Diagnosis

Most cases of hypothyroidism are diagnosed through medical blood lab testing. A doctor will order a thyroid panel that includes several tests or he will possibly order a single test. These tests will measure the T3 and/or T4 thyroid hormones levels and/or the TSH level (Thyroid Stimulating Hormone).

With hypothyroidism, the T3 and/or T4 levels will decrease to low levels, while the TSH will increase to a high level. This is due to TSH being the hormone as mentioned earlier, that stimulates hormone production in the thyroid gland and when the gland is not producing enough, the pituitary increases TSH to an abnormally high level. In some cases, TSH will be the test that detects hypothyroidism earlier than any other tests.

Less commonly used tests to detect hypothyroidism are the "Radioactive Iodine Scan" and the "Radioactive Iodine Uptake Test". The first mentioned scan is done by administering radioactive iodine to a patient and taking radiology camera images to see how evenly the thyroid gland is absorbing iodine. The second mentioned test does not involve imaging but is a measure of how much iodine is being absorbed by the thyroid gland.

If the thyroid gland fails to absorb an adequate amount of iodine, hypothyroidism may be diagnosed.

These tests are more commonly used to determine causes of hyperthyroidism (overactive gland) when excessive amounts of iodine are absorbed and to detect thyroid nodules (tumors) when iodine is absorbed unevenly in the gland.

Treatment

The goal of treatment for hypothyroidism is to increase low levels of thyroid hormone via a dose of prescribed replacement hormone. Doctors often prescribe synthetic T4 hormone drugs but some do prescribe combinations of T4 and T3 that come in either synthetic or natural brands. There is ongoing controversy in regard to which type of replacement hormone works best but the importance of the hypothyroid therapy lies in how well it is monitored and optimized.

The goal is to accomplish best possible symptom relief for patients, with dose adjustments made to restore bodily metabolism to the best possible level. This is done by monitoring the dose via repeat blood tests at approximately 8-week intervals, to measure the TSH, T4 and T3 levels. Once the proper levels are reached, TSH may be the only repeat blood test that is needed, with retests repeated about 2 to 4 times yearly.

In chapters that follow, more detail will be given to the subject of thyroid hormone replacement therapy, the treatment for cases of hypothyroidism.

CHAPTER TWO

Primary and Secondary Hypothyroid Disorders

Direct and Indirect Causes of an Underactive Thyroid Gland

Most cases of hypothyroidism are due to problems within the thyroid gland but there are other causes that indirectly cause under-functioning of the gland.

Thyroid disease is a primary cause of hypothyroidism, meaning it is a problem within the thyroid gland itself. Secondary causes of hypothyroidism would be those that do not originate within the gland but are other problems within the body that indirectly affect thyroid hormone levels.

Primary Causes

Thyroid autoimmunity - is an immune system response, in which auto-antibodies are created to attack thyroid proteins and is the most common cause of hypothyroidism in industrialized countries. In addition to causing destruction of thyroid tissue over time that result in the gland under-functioning, normal thyroid tissue is also taken over by abnormal tissue. Eventually, the gland can no longer absorb iodine from things in the diet, to produce thyroid hormone from.

This may also include development of thyroid nodules (small tumors) that take up space within the gland, so that there is less normal tissue for normal thyroid functioning.

Other primary causes – include injuries to the thyroid gland that diminish its ability to function normally and glands that are not fully developed at birth or following birth. If for example, a person is in a severe car accident that causes trauma to the throat, the thyroid gland can be directly damaged and once this occurs, any resulting hypothyroidism would be a problem within the gland. People who are born with only partial thyroid glands or small inadequate ones that do not develop as they become adults, can experience hypothyroidism which would also be a problem originating within the gland itself.

Secondary Causes

Biochemical hypothyroidism – are cases in which a chemical element needed by the thyroid gland is lacking or the gland is damaged by a drug or other chemical that is harmful to the body or hinders thyroid function. Iodine deficiency is in this category and occurs when there is inadequate iodine consumed in the diet. The thyroid is highly dependent on this chemical element that is used by the gland to produce hormones that regulate metabolism and so iodine deficiency causes the thyroid to hypo-function.

An example of chemical damage to the thyroid and resulting hypothyroidism would be when drinking water has been contaminated with radioactive chemicals and results in cell destruction within the gland.

Failure of major endocrine brain glands – is a condition often referred to as "Central Hypothyroidism", meaning the brain-center is failing to regulate the thyroid gland. The two master glands that stimulate the thyroid to operate at normal levels are the hypothalamus and pituitary glands. The hypothalamus sends TRH (thyrotrophin releasing hormone) to the pituitary gland, which in turn sends TSH (thyroid stimulating hormone), also called "thyrotrophin" to the thyroid gland, which completes the process by supplying the body with thyroid hormones. A failure on the part of either master gland, due to tumors within them or disease processes affecting them, results in secondary/central hypothyroidism.

Other secondary causes – include women who develop under-functioning thyroid glands as a result of pregnancy, also referred to as "postpartum hypothyroidism". Certain types of diseases can also affect thyroid function, including those affecting other glands in the endocrine system (hormone producing).

Chronic stress and severe emotional disorders can cause the T3 thyroid hormone specifically to become low. This less-common condition is referred to as "Euthyroid Sick Syndrome" or "low T3 Syndrome" and is a secondary cause that usually only requires short term treatment to resolve it.

Patients who are diagnosed with hypothyroidism should request that their doctors inform them of the cause of their thyroid disorder. This may require additional diagnostic testing but will help better-educate patients about the disease that is affecting them.

65

CHAPTER THREE

Hashimoto's Disease and Hypothyroid Treatment

Hypothyroidism from Autoimmune Thyroiditis

Hashimoto's is an autoimmune type of thyroiditis that leads to hypothyroidism. While there is no cure for the disease, the resulting hypothyroidism can be treated.

Hashimoto's thyroiditis affects approximately 14-million Americans and is 7 times more common in women than in men. It is the leading cause of hypothyroidism in industrialized countries and the second leading cause of an under-active thyroid gland in people worldwide, taking second place to iodine deficiency hypothyroidism. While there is no cure for this autoimmune thyroid disease, there is treatment for the hypothyroidism it causes.

Hashimoto's is an Autoimmune Disease

With Hashimoto's thyroiditis, auto-antibodies including the "anti-thyroidperoxidase" and the "anti-thyroglobulin" are created by the immune system to attack the thyroid gland. For reasons yet to be fully understood by medical research, the immune system will at times target a natural part of the body and will relentlessly attack it. There are a number of theories including viral agents, allergens or intolerant foods entering the body as causes of autoimmune responses.

Viruses that cannot be fully eliminated by the immune system for example may result in it turning on the body to destroy tissues that contain the virus. For whatever reason the body turns on itself with autoimmune diseases, it causes a mistaken identity. These natural tissues, organs, glands, muscles or joints are recognized as enemies in the body and are attacked. When the immune system is operating properly, it will create antibodies only to attack unnatural invaders that can potentially cause illness or disease in the body. With Hashimoto's, the immune system has turned on the thyroid gland to destroy it as a mistaken enemy.

Hashimoto's leads to Hypothyroidism

As the killer cells called "thyroid antibodies" begin to destroy natural thyroid gland protein-cells, it begins to cause death to the gland at a gradual rate. Antibody levels can vary among Hashimoto's patients and those with very high elevations of thyroid antibodies may see faster cell destruction and damage to the gland. As the damage occurs, the gland becomes less capable of producing thyroid hormone to regulate the metabolism of the body.

The resulting condition of slowed-metabolism is called "hypothyroidism". Many patients with the disease experience few or no symptoms until hypothyroidism begins to set in.

67

Mild cases of an under-active thyroid from
Hashimoto's can begin to cause symptoms of fatigue,
weight gain, fluid retention (myxedema), dry skin and
brittle hair, depression and/or anxiety and
constipation.

Treatment for Hashimoto's

This autoimmune thyroiditis is irreversible in the vast
majority of cases and medical research has not found
a cure for autoimmune diseases in-general nor do they
understand why they go into remission in rare cases.
The treatment that will need to be administered is for
the resulting hypothyroidism caused by the disease.
Once symptoms and/or lab tests reveal that the
thyroid gland has become under-active, thyroid
hormone replacement therapy is the treatment that is
administered.

Some medical sources also believe that hormone
replacement may help to reduce thyroid antibody
levels over time. Other medical research articles state
that supplementing Hashimoto's patients with
"selenium" may also help to reduce high elevations of
thyroid antibodies but the dose should be at a proper
level and monitored by a treating physician.

CHAPTER FOUR

Risks for Developing Hypothyroidism

Factors Contributing to an Underactive Thyroid Gland

There are genetic factors and other natural events that occur in life that place people at higher risk for the development of thyroid disease.

Thyroid diseases can affect anyone at any point in their lives there are however things that can add to the already present potential or probability that a person will develop a disease or disorder affecting thyroid hormone balance. With 80% of thyroid problems being in the hypothyroidism (under-functioning) category, this is the area that will be addressed in the following subheadings.

Being Female

If a person is female, rather than male, her chance for developing hypothyroidism has already increased at least five-fold. While statistics vary, it can be reasonably stated that thyroid disease in-general is no less than five times more common in women than in men. The female endocrine system (hormone producing) is more complicated than that of males due to there being the reproductive organs present, for giving birth.

These will experience the cycling each month from the age of puberty that signals times of high fertility (menses).

The fertility cycles that occur in females cause wide swings in the levels of sex, adrenal and thyroid hormones and may be the reason hormone imbalances and diseases develop more often affecting the endocrine systems of women. The endocrine system as a whole works in unison or what might be referred to as "a loop" or "in sync" and so changes in the levels of one endocrine hormone, can affect the levels of others.

It may be possible that these changes in endocrine hormones trigger an immune system response in some women (autoimmune disease), in which antibodies are created to attack the glands causing these wide fluctuations. When, the thyroid gland is affected it is referred to as "thyroid autoimmunity".

As women enter the age when reproduction responsiveness slows down (menopause), this too may contribute to thyroid hormone imbalance. Some medical sources are of the opinion that birth control pills may contribute to development of thyroid problems as well.

Being the Offspring of Parents with Thyroid Disease

If one or both of a person's parents have thyroid disease, this places him or her at high risk for developing thyroid problems of their own. According to Hossein Gharib, M.D., a member of the AACE (American Association of Clinical Endocrinologists) and a medical research professor at the Mayo Medical College, 50% of thyroid disorder parents will have offspring that inherit the gene responsible for thyroid disease development. Some medical sources state that thyroid problems can be present in children of thyroid disease parents, at birth or in early childhood but will not be detectable in most of them until about the age of 35 or 40 years.

Pregnancy

Approximately two percent of women, who become pregnant, develop under-active thyroid glands. Thyroid disorders during pregnancy can range from temporary thyroiditis to permanent hypothyroidism requiring lifelong treatment (25% are permanent). Thyroid disorders can manifest during pregnancy or following (postpartum) and estimates state that up to 10% of cases develop within a year after giving birth. Most cases involve under-active thyroid glands with only about 1% being cases of hyperthyroidism (overactive).

Senior Citizens

Generally, thyroid disease occurs most commonly in the general population at between the ages of 35 and 40. Those who do not develop thyroid problems due to other factors as detailed in the previous subheadings can still develop age-related hypothyroidism as they reach their senior years. Approximately 15% of women develop hypothyroidism by the age of 60 years and approximately 8% of men do so by the same age.

These cases are generally not due to a disease process but are a result of a diminished ability for thyroid glands in the elderly to produce the needed levels of hormones. Their glands are in-essence experiencing a degree of atrophy, meaning shrinkage and a diminished ability to function at pre-senior age levels. If thyroid symptoms do not appear in males or females by age 40, it is still recommended that blood testing of thyroid hormones be conducted to rule out developing thyroid disease.

CHAPTER FIVE

Varied Effectiveness of Thyroid Hormone Therapy

Optimized Treatment for Hypothyroidism

Hypothyroid patients deserve specialized treatment from treating doctors who monitor and adjust their thyroid hormone dose to best possible symptom-relieving levels.

For patients with hypothyroidism, thyroid hormone replacement therapy effectiveness is very important. The more symptom relief that can be experienced, the better patients are able to carry on normal activities of work, school and leisure activities. In other words, they will regain the best quality-of-life possible. This is where the importance in securing the best possible doctor for administering the treatment comes in, as well as his or her ability to best optimize that therapy.

The fact is, that thyroid hormone therapies vary in effectiveness, depending upon the type that is being administered and how well it is being monitored by the treating doctor via repeat blood lab testing. Most hypothyroid patients need dose adjustments to bring their thyroid hormones back to the proper level and eventually finely-tuned further to an optimal level.

Each patient has that target level that brings them the most symptom relief or what might be called their "set-point".

This level of treatment varies among patients and further demonstrates the importance in a quality thyroid doctor, meaning one who specializes in optimizing treatment for hypothyroid patients.

Finding the Right Type of Thyroid Hormone Dose

Most patients are started on a dose of thyroxine to treat their hypothyroidism, which is a T4 only hormone dose, usually prescribed in the synthetic form. The two major thyroid hormones that regulate the body's metabolism are the T4 and T3 and we depend on the body's natural process of converting the needed T3 from the T4. For some patients this does not happen adequately and this problem is referred to as "impaired conversion".

The treating doctor also needs to be aware of these possibilities and to know how to monitor for them. If a patient does experience impaired conversion, the doctor needs to be willing to add T3 hormone to the patient's replacement therapy dose. Some doctors start patients on T4/T3 combination hormone doses because they believe it is more effective in some patients than a T4-only dose.

The Importance of Repeat Blood Test Monitoring

To fully monitor the hormone therapy of newly treated hypothyroid patients, a doctor needs to order full thyroid panels.

74

This would include TSH, T4 and T3, the "free levels" of the later two being the better versions (as opposed to the "total levels") according to many thyroid specialists and endocrinologists. This more thorough monitoring for at least the first few blood retests will better evaluate the thyroid hormone therapy and help the doctor to know what changes are needed in the dose or type of thyroid hormone that is needed.

If this type of specialized treatment is not offered to hypothyroid patients, many may potentially remain in a state of unrelieved hypothyroid symptoms and the opportunity will be missed to restore a better quality-of-life to them.

CHAPTER SIX

T4 and T3 Hypothyroid Treatment Options

Hormone Treatments for an Underactive Thyroid

Some hypothyroid patients are successfully treated with a T4 thyroid hormone replacement dose. Others may also need T3 hormone added to their treatment.

The majority of diagnosed hypothyroid patients are prescribed T4 replacement hormone medications. These are types/brands that replace low thyroxine levels, which is the T4 hormone that also converts into the other major thyroid hormone called T3 (triiodothyronine). Brands of thyroxine are also referred to as "levothyroxine sodium" and include the following brands.

• Synthroid

• Levoxyl

• Levothroid

• Unithroid

Thyroxine-T4 Replacement Therapy and Impaired Conversion

Once a dose of T4-only replacement hormone is taken, the treated patient and treating doctor must depend on the T4 to successfully convert into T3 as it is needed in the body.

In the majority of hypothyroid patients, this occurs adequately as needed; however, in a small percent of patients, they will experience "impaired conversion". The lack of T3 being converted will keep them in a state of hypothyroidism or what might be referred to as "Low T3 Syndrome". Monitoring for impaired conversion requires the treating doctor to retest the patient's blood levels of both T4 and T3 to see if proper conversion is occurring. This phenomenon will be mentioned further in chapters that follow.

Combination T4 and T3 Replacement Therapy

Some doctors, who treat hypothyroidism, prefer to prescribe combination T4 and T3 thyroid hormone replacement medications. They believe this type of therapy is superior to T4-only replacement whether impaired conversion is an issue or not. Brands of combination T4 and T3 thyroid hormone drugs include the following.

• Thyrolar

• Armour Thyroid

• Nature-Throid

• Westhroid

Most cases of hypothyroidism are caused by types of "thyroid autoimmunity", also referred to as chronic thyroiditis (i.e. Hashimoto's, Riedel's and Ord's).

Auto-antibodies sent from the immune system, to attack thyroid proteins that convert iodine into thyroid hormones. Because of this, there can be a significant percent of hormone being blocked from conversion and this will cause the T3 level to remain at sub-optimal level, even when the dose of T4 coming into the body is adequate. While the T3 may remain within normal range, it will stay slightly below the mid-level of normal values or at lower normal.

The Treatment Goal for T4 and T3

Some hypothyroid patients may experience better symptom relief if both the T4 and T3 are at mid-range or higher-normal. This can be accomplished in most patients who are placed on a T4-only dose but for those whose ratio of T4 to T3 is not remaining balanced at mid-range or above, a combination of T4 and T3 thyroid hormone dose may offer the solution. This too is better determined by testing both thyroid hormone levels in treated hypothyroid patients. Testing the TSH alone (Thyroid Stimulating Hormone) may not detect a low T3 level in some cases either. This pituitary gland hormone may test at normal range even if the T4-only is at proper level but the T3 is not.

Triiodothyronine-T3 Replacement Therapy

A dose of T3-only (Liothyronine Sodium) is usually restricted to cases of "Low T3 Syndrome".

This is what is also commonly referred to as "Euthyroid Sick Syndrome" or "Wilson's Syndrome". This condition of low T3 can occur in heart disease patients, in athletes who undergo strenuous training and in people with severe depression or chronic stress. It can also occur in cancer patients and in other cases of chronic or inflammatory diseases. A T3 dose of thyroid hormone replacement may be administered to patients with this type of hypothyroidism caused by low T3 levels. The cause of the hypothyroidism will also be treated or corrected and if significant improvement occurs, the T3 replacement therapy may only be needed temporarily (short-term).

Doses of T3-only hormone medications are also sometimes added to T4 doses in hypothyroid patients so that the treating doctor can choose the specific ratio of T4 to T3 he deems necessary for the patient. The most recognized brand of T3 hormone available is called "Cytomel", manufactured by King Pharmaceuticals. Some doctors may also refer their hypothyroid patients to compounding pharmacies who combine the needed ratio of T4 to T3 into a specially manufactured dose, tailored to the individual patient's needs.

CHAPTER SEVEN

Hypothyroid Therapy Adjustment Symptoms

Thyroid Hormone Replacement Side Effects

Some patients who start hormone replacement therapy for hypothyroidism will experience adjustment symptoms to the new dose.

Most newly treated hypothyroid patients see these adjustment symptoms resolve after a few weeks on their thyroid medication. Many patients require one or more dose increases following an initial starting dose to elevate their thyroid hormone levels to a proper level. This process can take several months before an adequate or optimal treatment level is achieved.

How Doctors Monitor Treatment

A new dose is monitored via follow up blood retests as previously mentioned and if it is found to be lower than is needed to adequately treat a patient's hypothyroidism, it is increased. In some cases a dose increase may be needed several times to reach the desired level and in some cases a dose decrease may be needed (a lower dose) if levels test abnormally high at some point.

Several months between a scheduled blood retest, a patient may experience symptoms that indicate the need for a dose adjustment.

The treating doctor may retest the levels earlier than scheduled in this case and adjust the patient's dose accordingly.

If a patient's dose is too low, they may experience one or more of the following hypothyroid symptoms:

• constipation

• depression

• fatigue

• excessive need for sleep

• dry skin

• joint and muscle aches

If a patient's dose is too high, they may experience hyperthyroid symptoms that include the following:

• rapid heart rate

• diarrhea

• anxiety and nervousness

• sweating

• tremors

• insomnia

• muscle weakness

Types of Thyroid Hormone Doses

Adjustment symptoms may occur more often in patients who take replacement hormone brands that contain the T3 thyroid hormone (it is at least five times more potent that T4); however, patients who take a T4-only hormone may also experience dose-adjustment type symptoms. It takes approximately eight weeks to see a new dose level-out in the body and to start doing it's job properly.

The following are types of prescribed thyroid hormone medications that are administered to hypothyroid patients and that require adjustment to them in the body.

• synthetic T4

• synthetic T3

• combination synthetic T4 and T3

•combination natural (animal derived) T4 and T3

• compounded (varied ratio) mix of T4 and T3

How the Thyroid Gland Responds to Replacement Therapy

Many patients, who do experience adjustment type symptoms to thyroid hormone replacement, will either see worsening hypothyroid symptoms or may have some mild to moderate hyperthyroid type symptoms. Either type usually resolves after a few weeks.

This happens because the thyroid gland responds to hormone coming into the body from the outside, by shutting off part or all of its own production of hormone. When this happens, the body sometimes reaches a break-even point before improvement of hypothyroid symptoms begins.

Other patient's thyroid glands are slower to cut back production of hormone, as the dose comes into the body, so will experience hyperthyroid type symptoms for a brief period of time. These two scenarios can also depend on how much damage has occurred in the thyroid gland from antibody-destruction, meaning the attack from auto-antibodies being sent to the gland from the immune system (thyroid autoimmunity).

If a patient's thyroid gland has been damaged from highly elevated antibody levels, as a dose of thyroid hormone is administered, their own gland will begin shutting down (atrophy) and adjustment symptoms may occur in the body. This might also be referred to as "side effects" from the starting dose.

Suppressing the TSH Level

According to the U.S. NIH (National Institutes of Health) a hormone replacement dose for hypothyroidism needs to suppress the blood TSH level (pituitary hormone that reflects thyroid levels) down to between 0.5 and 3.0 mIU/L over time (average TSH normal range: 0.5 to 5.0 mIU/L).

The T4 and T3 need to be raised to around mid-range or upper-normal (ranges vary among testing labs).

This can take time and possibly several dose adjustments monitored at eight-week intervals by blood retests of TSH, T4 & T3. Most doctors prefer to start patients on a low dose and increase it upward (titrate) until it reaches the proper level to sufficiently treat a patient's hypothyroidism.

CHAPTER EIGHT

Distinguishing between Diagnostic and Treatment TSH

A Narrower Normal Values Range for Treating Hypothyroidism

The normal reference range for Thyroid Stimulating Hormone (diagnostic TSH) is not the same as the range used by most doctors for treating under active thyroid glands.

The goal of thyroid hormone therapy to treat patients with hypothyroid conditions is to suppress their elevated TSH levels, down to a lower normal level. As the TSH is suppressed, the thyroid hormone levels (T4 and T3) will rise in response to corrected levels (from low to normal). Keeping TSH at a higher normal level, even if that level remains within normal values, may not result in adequate treatment for some patients.

Diagnostic TSH Range

The normal values TSH range for detecting thyroid hormone imbalance at medical blood labs has a high-normal boundary and a low-normal boundary. Readings falling outside of those, even slightly, can indicate an existing thyroid hormone imbalance or one that is developing.

The range will be fairly wide, so that less-than borderline cases do not appear to be abnormal readings, which can be misleading to a doctor, resulting in additional testing or follow-up monitoring that may not be necessary.

A blood lab for example may have a normal range for TSH, to diagnose thyroid dysfunction that is from 0.4 to 4.0, with readings that fall below 0.4 indicating thyroid hormone levels are elevating in the body and with readings rising above 4.0 indicating thyroid hormones are decreasing in the body. If readings are at either of the cut-off levels but not outside of them (borderline), these cases still merit follow up retesting because they may point to developing thyroid hormone imbalance. This is a fact stated by the U.S. National Institutes of Health.

Treatment TSH Range

When hypothyroidism is being treated, which can develop directly from a disease process or following treatment for hyperthyroidism, the goal is not simply to correct the TSH level back into the normal values range. The goal is rather to treat the hypothyroidism, so that TSH is at a level that also places the thyroid hormones at the proper level to relieve symptoms of hypothyroidism and to correct the patient's slow functioning metabolism.

A borderline high or higher-normal TSH level may not accomplish this; in fact some patients may require TSH to be suppressed to low-normal levels to properly increase the T4 and T3. Blood testing all three levels together can better help to determine where the TSH level needs to be.

TSH Range - Too wide at Some Labs

Both the AACE (American Association of Clinical Endocrinologists) and the NACB (National Academy of Clinical Biochemistry) have recommended that labs with wide TSH ranges, narrow those ranges to a level that detects more cases of developing thyroid hormone disorders. The AACE has expressed belief that TSH levels above "3.0" may indicate developing hypothyroidism, while the NACB states that the upper limit (high normal) TSH reference range may at some point need to be reduced to "2.5". This is based on their observance of the fact that 95% of euthyroid (normal thyroid function) individuals test between "0.4 and 2.5".

CHAPTER NINE

Thyroid Hormone Treatment Controversies

Issues of Debate Regarding Hypothyroid Therapies

The debate is ongoing as to which type hormone replacement therapy is best. The answer is not actually a "one size fits all" one but one of patient-individuality.

Doctors who treat hypothyroidism should see each patient as an individual who needs monitored for both the effectiveness of the treatment and possible problems that might arise from the thyroid hormone replacement therapy. If a patient fails to experience satisfactory symptom relief, a trial of a different type of prescribed hormone might hold the answer to better treatment success.

Brand Favoritism In-Balance

Doctors should certainly form their opinions as to which thyroid hormone type or brand works better in the general population of hypothyroid patients. When a doctor however, highly favors a particular brand over all others, to the point of unwillingness to switch patients struggling with unresolved symptoms to trials of other types, this could result in missed opportunities for improved symptom-relief for individual patients who sometimes have unique treatment-needs.

Doctors should also be willing to consider suggestions by their patients, as to which thyroid hormone therapy they feel might be better suited for them. All available types require being prescribed by a treating doctor who will also monitor the treatment and a preference expressed by a patient for a particular type or brand does not change this fact. Doctors, who do not specialize in thyroid treatment or who are having problems treating patients with difficult cases, should also be willing to refer them to Thyroid Specialists or Endocrinologists when needed.

Does Synthetic T4 Restore Metabolism?

There has been very strong debate by advocates on both sides of the thyroid hormone brand issue, one being represented by proponents who feel natural brands of T4 and T3 combination are the best treatment-option for hypothyroidism, the other being proponents who believe synthetic T4-only to be the best treatment-option. Points that are often included in the debate include the view that both T4 and T3 are needed to restore normal metabolism in many hypothyroid patients.

In defense of thyroxine-only replacement therapy (not containing T3), it is often pointed out that once a proper dose-level of synthetic T4 is administered, the proof of how well the hormone is being used by the body can be seen in follow-up blood tests.

These tests and retests can include one that also measures the Free T3 level which can determine if the patient's body is properly recognizing the hormone and converting it into the proper level of this more metabolically active hormone.

The other consideration is "symptom improvement" (including correction of elevated cholesterol levels) and if both of these factors are satisfactorily taking place, why would a patient or doctor want to see the type or brand of treatment switched? Trying to fix things that are not broken can sometimes cause more problems than solutions.

"T3 Does Not Add Benefit for Some Patients."

This type statement fits into the "one size fits all" category of debate-view and while it may be true in some cases it will not be true in all cases. One aspect that is often added to this argument against the addition of T3 hormone into a treatment for a hypothyroid patient is the fact that the hormone is fast-acting and has a shorter half-life than T4 has. The opinion therefore is that it is unstable in patients and causes spikes and crashes in T3 levels. The fact is however that treatment containing T3 is taken on a daily basis and this alone helps to keep levels stable.

Additionally, the same mentions in the previous subheading in regard to blood retests that monitor thyroid hormone replacement therapy also apply to therapies that include T3.

Hypothyroidism-The Best Darn Complete Look

If blood levels remain stable and symptom-relief is experienced, this should signal treatment success to both the patient and doctor.

There are also medical studies that have concluded that hypothyroid therapy in depressed patients with difficult to resolve depression symptoms, can benefit from the addition of T3 to their thyroid hormone replacement therapy. This too is a factor demonstrating patient-individuality and another consideration both patient and doctor should look at if this scenario involving depression exists in a patient.

Allergies and Intolerances

A small percent of patients placed on certain types of thyroid hormone whether synthetic or natural brands will have allergic or intolerant reactions to them. Many medications contain fillers that help manufactures process them into pill form or that help the drug to better absorb in the systems of patients who take them. These patients, whose systems recognize these fillers as allergens, will experience symptoms such as hives and stomach upset. This will require the treating doctor to switch the patient to a brand that is better tolerated.

Some thyroid hormone brands are derived from the glands of pigs (porcine source) and there are people who are intolerant to any type of pork or related products.

In cases like these it may be either the synthetic or the natural brand that works better for these patients with sensitivities. Some natural brands of thyroid hormone are "hypoallergenic", meaning all know allergy-causing ingredients have been removed.

Generic Vs Major Brands

Some patients will see their doctors change their prescriptions from a major thyroid hormone brand, to a generic for insurance purposes or to save self-pay patients on their costs. Generics in all types of medications have been found to sometimes be slightly less potent when compared to major brands. In the case of thyroid hormone therapy, this can mean that the patient's T4 and T3 levels may drop slightly as a result of switching to a generic brand. This will require the treating doctor to increase the dose level to compensate for the different in potency.

With any switch of a thyroid hormone prescription, whether from synthetic to natural or from major brand to generic, patients need blood retested about eight weeks following the switch-over. If blood retesting is set at a longer interval of three to six months, the patient may experience a period of hypothyroid symptoms.

Additional Reasons for Brand Preferences

In addition to the aforementioned, there are other reasons some patients require a particular brand of thyroid hormone or who must be restricted from certain brands. Some patients for example, experience a less-common condition called "low T3 syndrome" that requires replacing only the T3 thyroid hormone until the condition resolves. The reverse can also be true, demonstrated by the fact that some hypothyroid patients are highly sensitive to T3 supplementation. They will have hyperthyroid type side effects from even low doses of oral dosing which in some cases may be due to another type of deficiency or hormone imbalance present in their bodies.

In other cases, a person's religious beliefs or convictions restrict the use of products made from certain animals. This can also be true of people who practice firm beliefs in the area of animal advocacy or who, are vegetarians. All of the preceding described reasons demonstrate the reasons for the existence of synthetic, natural and variation of T4 and T3 brands.

CHAPTER TEN

Optimizing Hypothyroidism Treatment Levels

TSH Monitoring of Thyroid Hormone Therapy

Most treated hypothyroid patients experience significant symptom relief and regain normal metabolism, while others experience difficulties with inadequate treatment.

Thyroid hormone replacement is simple to administer and requires that a patient take a daily dose of synthetic or natural thyroid hormone to restore bodily metabolism. While the method of treatment is simple, it is also important that a treating doctor is sensitive to the needs of individual patients. This demonstrates the importance in hypothyroid patients being treated by qualified thyroid doctors and in patients being fully communicative about progress and symptom-relief (or a lack in these) with their treating doctors.

Optimized Treatment Goals

It is a fact that there are doctors who specialize in thyroid treatments and those who do not. Those who do often have targeted treatment goals for patients, rather than simply treating them to get their thyroid hormone levels replaced back into the normal values range. The two major thyroid hormones that are monitored with hypothyroid therapy are the T4 and T3 levels.

A low-normal thyroid hormone level or even one that is at about mid-range will not be optimal for some patients who instead need the levels at between mid-range and high-normal to experience significant symptom relief.

TSH Suppression

Looking at it from the point-of-view of the TSH level (pituitary hormone that reflects thyroid hormone levels), the goal of a replacement thyroid hormone dose is to suppress the elevated TSH level (elevates with hypothyroidism) back down to normal range. Some patients however, need a significantly suppressed TSH to cause thyroid hormones (T4 and T3) to rise slightly above mid-range in the body.

If the TSH normal values range at a blood lab is for example from "0.5 to 5.0IU/L", a thyroid hormone dose that only suppresses TSH down to "3.5" may not result in adequate increases in thyroid hormone levels or in the symptom relief that is needed by the patient. The U.S. National Institutes of Health states that hypothyroidism should be treated to place a patient's TSH level at between "0.5 and 3.0 mIU/L". Levels such as "1.0" and "2.0" are within that treatment goal range.

Patient Individuality

The scenario addressed in the previous subheading is
sometimes reversed and a hypothyroid patient may
not need a significantly suppressed TSH for thyroid
hormone levels to become optimized. Some patients
in fact will experience mild, ongoing hyperthyroid
(overactive) type symptoms if their TSH is
suppressed below a "2.5" or "2.0". It is not always
apparent as to why patients may vary in this area but
could be due to differences in the functioning of their
regulating brain glands (the master endocrine ones),
or more specifically in how their pituitary function
may vary slightly in response to thyroid hormone
coming into the body from an outside source (the
resulting TSH level).

Blood Retesting TSH and Thyroid Hormones

Detecting differences in the needs of individual
patients may require blood testing their T4 and T3
levels in addition to TSH, to better evaluate how these
levels all correlate. Once a doctor knows where the
TSH level needs to fall within the treatment range to
optimize a patient's thyroid hormone levels via a
replacement dose, he can then blood retest using
TSH-only. If TSH and thyroid hormones are not first
evaluated together in follow up on hypothyroid
therapy, opportunity to better optimize a patient's
treatment might be missed.

CHAPTER ELEVEN

Thyroid Disease Related Depression

When Thyroid Treatment does not Relieve Depression

Thyroid treatments do not always successfully resolve the emotional symptoms of depression in all patients. Some need additional treatments or therapies administered.

Thyroid hormone imbalances are well-known for causing emotional and mood disorders including major depression. Both hypothyroid and hyperthyroid conditions have potential to cause symptoms of depression and/or anxiety. For some well-treated thyroid patients, their emotional symptoms persist and they need additional help with coping and symptom relief, through added medications or therapies.

Symptoms of Depression

People who become depressed will experience extreme sadness that is profound and not always related to a traumatic or life-altering event. The already-present depression can worsen however, if such events occur, such as the loss of a loved one, change in careers or moving to a new location, away from friends and family.

Depression also causes a loss of ability to enjoy things that were once pleasurable or to become motivated by things that were previously of interest. Depressed people often have a lack of energy and will feel fatigued and a need to sleep more than the average person not suffering from depression. For thyroid patients, thyroid hormone imbalance can directly cause or contribute to worsening depression.

Adequate Thyroid Treatment

When depression persists in thyroid patients who are being treated, the first and most important thing to consider is whether the treatment is adequate. A person who is diagnosed with hypothyroidism for example and hyperthyroid patients who become hypothyroid after surgical removal or ablation of their thyroid glands (thyroidectomy or radioactive iodine destruction), need to be adequately treated with thyroid hormone replacement therapy. If their dose is not at a level that fully restores their metabolism, they may remain in a state of unresolved symptoms, including those of depression.

Some thyroid specializing doctors and endocrinologists set a goal for TSH of from about 1.0 to 2.0 to start with as mentioned previously. They may increase the dose to suppress TSH further, staying within normal values once adequate time is given to see if satisfactory symptom relief is achieved but is still not occurring.

Even small increases in dose can make a difference in how the patient responds to treatment, including improvement in depressed mood. Some doctors will also retest the actual thyroid hormone levels - T4 and T3, in addition to TSH to make sure the levels all correlate properly before considering additional drug or psychiatric treatment therapies.

Other Treatment Options for Depressed Thyroid Patients

As stated previously, research studies of hypothyroid patients have concluded that treatment-resistant depression is better resolved in some patients if a thyroid hormone replacement dose contains "T3 hormone" and not T4 only. There are brands of T3 thyroid hormone available and it is available already combined with T4. A treating doctor may be willing to prescribe a trial of T3 in treated patients who retain depression symptoms if they feel they are proper candidates for it (i.e. they are not hyper-sensitive to oral T3).

When best thyroid hormone treatment options have been tried and depression still persists, patients may need to be prescribed anti-depressant medications or referred for psychiatric therapies. In cases of severe depression, these added options may need to be administered immediately.

A highly successful psychiatric therapy used to treat both anxiety and depression, is one called "Cognitive Behavioral Therapy". A class of antidepressant drugs called Selective Serotonin Reuptake Inhibitors (SSRIs) has also proven to be effective in many cases of depression and/or anxiety conditions. Some patients may find significant symptom-relief from a combination of drug and psychiatric therapies and may respond favorably enough over time, so that they can slowly wean off of one or both treatments, under close supervision of their treating doctor(s).

CHAPTER TWELVE

Subclinical Hypothyroidism Treatment Challenges

Treating Mild Underactive Thyroid Conditions

Subclinical hypothyroidism is a term meaning an under-active thyroid gland is not at full-blown level (overt) and knowing when to treat these cases can be difficult for doctors.

Some hypothyroid patients experience significant symptoms even when their diagnostic blood labs indicate that their thyroid hormones are only mildly deficient. In these type cases, symptoms should be a consideration in deciding whether or not to begin thyroid hormone replacement therapy as well as determining if the patient has thyroid autoimmunity causing their condition. If auto-antibodies are the cause, starting treatment can help prevent antibodies from further increasing and causing further inflammation in the gland which can contribute to goiter (thyroid gland swelling) and other potential symptoms in the body.

Mild Hypothyroidism Detected by TSH

Most cases of subclinical hypothyroidism are revealed by an elevated TSH level (Thyroid Stimulating Hormone). This pituitary hormone, coming from the brain-gland, regulating thyroid function.

It increases to abnormally high levels when thyroid hormones begin to decrease (onset of hypothyroidism). The thyroid hormones, T4 and T3 will at the same time, fall within normal values, although they may be at lower-normal or even borderline-low.

Regardless of where the actual thyroid hormones fall within the normal range, if TSH is elevated even slightly above normal, this usually indicates that the thyroid gland is struggling to produce normal amounts of thyroid hormone to supply the body for maintaining normal metabolism. At this point, most patients do not experience noticeable symptoms, while a small percent of them do experience them and for some, symptoms can be significant. Another factor in whether symptoms are beginning depends on how close a sub clinical case is to becoming full-blown, or what is sometimes referred to as "overt hypothyroidism".

What TSH Level Merits Treating Hypothyroidism?

This question has led to some controversy in medical circles because there are two concerns involved with this issue. One being, that not treating sub clinical cases of hypothyroidism can lead to elevated cholesterol levels, contributing to heart disease over time.

The other being, that by treating early, when a patient does not yet fully need replacement thyroid hormone administered, it could induce mild thyrotoxicity (abnormal elevations in thyroid hormones). If treatment does cause mild hyperthyroidism in a patient, it can contribute to osteoporosis and arrhythmias in the heart (abnormal beats).

Some doctors want to see the TSH level elevated to a "10.0" or above before they begin treating hypothyroidism if thyroid hormones continue to stay within normal range. The AACE (American Association of Clinical Endocrinologists) however recently published recommendations in the year 2002, encouraging doctors to consider treating patients whose TSH levels reach levels above "3.04". They also recommended narrowing the diagnostic TSH range to "0.3 to 3.0" which will detect more cases of developing thyroid hormone disorders.

Symptoms and Thyroid Autoimmunity

If a patient with sub clinical hypothyroidism tests positive for thyroid antibodies, this may prompt a doctor to begin treatment due to the fact that thyroid autoimmunity increases the rate of progression to overt hypothyroidism. Some cases of mild under-active thyroid glands are age-related or may have no apparent cause and these can remain in a mild state, not causing symptoms.

These cases may not require treatment but will simply need to be monitored closely by blood retests of thyroid levels once or twice yearly.

If symptoms are present in mildly hypothyroid patients, this should be a consideration by doctors monitoring these cases because symptoms can affect quality-of-life in these patients. If additional blood testing reveals elevated cholesterol levels in these patients, this is an important consideration as well because treating with thyroid hormone replacement may be less difficult than treating with cholesterol lowering drugs (statins) which can produce a variety of potential side effects.

CHAPTER THIRTEEN

Best Thyroid Hormone Blood Tests

Diagnostic and Treatment Medical Lab Testing

There are a variety of tests used to both detect thyroid hormone imbalances and to monitor the treatments for them.

Which blood test is best depends on each individual case and depends on factors such as whether the case involves diagnosing thyroid hormone imbalance or if it is follow-up on treatment to correct a problem.

TSH the Most Sensitive Test

Thyroid Stimulating Hormone (TSH) is a pituitary gland hormone as previously mentioned, which is sent from the brain-center or what might be referred to as the "central command post" that monitors and regulates the amount of thyroid hormone released from the thyroid gland. It increases when the thyroid needs to produce more hormone and it decreases when it needs to produce less but in a non-diseased thyroid gland, these fluctuations stay within normal values. When hypothyroidism (under-active thyroid) or hyperthyroidism (overactive thyroid) occurs, TSH will begin to fall outside of the normal values range.

Because of how finely-tuned TSH keeps the thyroid gland, it will change its level in the body with even to most subtle changes in thyroid function.

If for example the thyroid becomes less able to provide adequate hormone in the body due to damage in the gland from a disease process affecting it, TSH will increase in level before thyroid hormones decrease in levels. It will continue to increase to higher levels as the thyroid becomes unable to supply normal amounts. During its attempt to keep the thyroid going at normal speed, the TSH hormone will first become mildly abnormal on blood lab tests. This makes TSH the single best and earliest indicator of developing thyroid hormone imbalance that is available.

Free T4 and Free T3

The T3 and T4 thyroid hormone levels can be tested as the "total" levels or as the "free" levels. Many thyroid specialists and endocrinologists believe that the free levels are the better blood tests. This is due to the fact that patients, who are undergoing cortisol steroid treatments for example or estrogen therapy or have certain medical conditions such as liver disease or pregnancy, can experience a change in the level of a thyroid protein called TBG (thyroxine-binding globulin). Much of the T3 is bound in the blood by this protein (total level) with the free, unbound T3 that is left over, being more active in regulating bodily metabolism. This is why some thyroid specialists prefer to test the free unbound levels.

Certain types of scenarios can change the free-circulating level of remaining T3 hormone in the body that is available including cases of thyroid disease. Depending on each particular case, this can result in Total T3 testing normal, while the Free T3 will test outside of normal values, better detecting thyroid hormone imbalances in some cases.

These two thyroid hormones (T3 and T4) are tested both to detect thyroid hormone imbalances and to monitor replacement hormone therapies. They are also sometimes tested to monitor thyroid hormone levels in hyperthyroid patients who have received treatment to slow down abnormally high thyroid hormone production or to retest their levels after they have had their thyroid glands removed as a treatment procedure.

Often, TSH is added to the Free T3 and Free T4 for a more thorough evaluation of patients because TSH alone will not always detect all types of thyroid hormone disorders, such as those caused by a problem within the thyroid-regulating brain glands rather than a problem within the thyroid gland itself.

Thyroid Panels

These groupings of tests, are ordered to better evaluate patients being diagnosed and will include both TSH and thyroid hormone levels (T3 and/or T4). A thyroid panel is often a better diagnostic tool than is TSH alone or a single thyroid hormone level.

This is because of factors including those discussed in the previous subheadings in which a thyroid hormone problem can be either primary (within the gland) or secondary (outside of the gland).

This can also be true of thyroid hormone therapies in which TSH alone is not accurate in monitoring treatment due to regulating brain gland problems or due to a problem with only one thyroid hormone level rather than both. The need for varied tests or for more thorough types of thyroid blood tests can occur with "Low T3 Syndromes" or in cases of "impaired conversion of T4 into T3" that is experienced by some thyroid patients taking T4 only replacement hormone medications.

CHAPTER FOURTEEN

Things That Affect Thyroid Hormones in the Body

Facts Treated Thyroid Patients Need to Know

With treated hypothyroidism the therapy is a "set dose" of thyroid hormone replacement. Patients need to be aware of things that can affect thyroid hormone levels in the body.

When a person's own thyroid gland is supplying hormone to the body, the levels will fluctuate as there is a need for them to do so. The pituitary gland in the brain regulates the amount of thyroid hormone released via stimulation of the thyroid gland by Thyroid Stimulating Hormone - TSH.

With thyroid hormone replacement therapy to treat an under active thyroid gland, the dose administered remains steady in the body and does not fluctuate due to things that might change the amount of hormone that is needed. This fact demonstrates the need by treated hypothyroid patients to know what things in their diets and lifestyle practices can affect thyroid hormone levels in the body.

Hard Physical Exercise

While exercise has many benefits, both physical and emotional, hard physical activity can have a lowering affect on thyroid hormone levels.

It is important for hypothyroid patients to pace their exercise regimens, so that they do not exceed their tolerance level because thyroid hormones will not rise to meet the extra demand when a set-dose is being taken. The resulting effect can be severe fatigue and slow recovery from hard physical activity. Exercise should be built upon slowly to a reasonable level and afterward maintained at the proper level, so that a thyroid hormone dose remains adequate, reflected in follow up blood retests that monitor the dose.

Alcohol, Caffeine and Smoking

Medical research studies have shown that alcohol consumption can negatively affect thyroid hormone levels and is especially true in pregnant women who can cause thyroid function to drop in both their own bodies and that of their fetuses with alcohol use. Alcohol acts as both a stimulant and a depressant and it could be that there are increases in thyroid hormones with alcohol use in smaller amounts that are followed by decreases in the levels with increased or prolonged alcohol use.

Another stimulant that has been shown to alter thyroid hormone production, is caffeine and medical studies done with animal models have shown that caffeine consumption temporarily increases thyroid hormone levels.

This might cause a temporary increase in energy as well but as with any stimulant, will also cause a resulting crash when levels drop back down to normal levels. Hypothyroid patients feel these fluctuations more intensely than do people with normal thyroid function whose bodies can adjust the thyroid hormone levels in response to these type influences.

A third stimulant that has also been studied by medical research groups but in this case using human models, is tobacco smoking. Studies have shown that smokers have elevated thyroid hormone levels and decreased TSH levels. Some of the conclusions in these studies state that smokers have a three-fold increased risk for developing Graves' disease, the autoimmune-cause of hyperthyroidism (overactive).

In hypothyroid patients with Hashimoto's thyroiditis (autoimmune cause), smoking may place them at higher risk for episodes of Hashitoxicosis (hyperthyroid phases) or for transitioning over to Graves' disease. A substantial risk that has been confirmed in medical research is the fact that smoking increases chances for the development of "Thyroid Eye Disease" (inflammatory condition) in autoimmune thyroid disorder patients.

Goitrogen Foods

It is a well known fact that eating foods high in calcium and/or iron or taking supplements containing these elements can hinder absorption of a thyroid hormone dose, unless taken at least four hours apart from the dose (some sources recommend six hours). There are, however other foods that can actually cause thyroid hormone levels to decrease, regardless of when eaten, called "goitrogens". These type foods are medically recognized for their ability to lower thyroid hormone levels in the body due to their effect in blocking the action of "thyroid peroxidase" (protein/enzyme).

One major food group well-known for its thyroid hormone diminishing ability is soy products. Reading ingredient labels can reveal which products contain soy apart from the obvious ones. Other foods that can have a goitrogenic affect are those from the cruciferous family of vegetables.

These include

• mustard

• rutabaga

• turnips

• broccoli

• brussel sprouts

- cabbage

- cauliflower

- kale

- kohlrabi

- spinach

- radishes

Nuts, grains and fruits in the goitrogen category include the following:

- millet

- peanuts

- soybeans

- strawberries

- peaches

Treated hypothyroid patients should avoid these foods beyond small servings (large portions) and thoroughly cooking them can help diminish their goitrogenic effects.

CHAPTER FIFTEEN

Thyroid Symptoms May Need Special Attention

When Hormone Replacement Does Not Give Adequate Symptom Relief

While most symptoms are relieved with treatments designed for thyroid hormone imbalances there are some common problem-symptoms that treated patients commonly experience.

The symptoms addressed in this article can also be those that require additional attention by the patient and/or the treating doctor, if thyroid treatment alone does not satisfactorily alleviate them.

Fatigue

This symptom often not relieved satisfactorily in treated thyroid patients may be the number one problem affecting them, according to some surveys. It is also a strong possibility that fatigue is associated with thyroid autoimmunity (the disease process) and not a result of abnormal thyroid hormone levels alone. In addition to Fibromyalgia being commonly suspected in thyroid patients before they receive definitive diagnoses of thyroid problems, they are also commonly suspected of having Chronic Fatigue Syndrome (CFS) before proper blood testing reveals thyroid hormone abnormalities.

Some patients after being well-treated and that have had all other possible causes of fatigue ruled-out, may receive a diagnosis of CFS being co-morbid (co-occurring) with thyroid disease.

The U.S. Centers for Disease Control now recognizes the fact that thyroid disease can co-exist with CFS and other medical studies conclude that autoimmune diseases of any kind may serve as a trigger for causing CFS. Things that can help patients who continue experiencing fatigue despite proper thyroid treatment, would include supplementing with Vitamins B5, B5, B6, B12, C and E, folic acid, CoQ10 and the herbal remedies called ginkgo biloba and ginseng. These supplements have been found to increase cellular energy in the body and may help to increase oxygen levels in the blood.

A patient should inform their doctor when taking any new supplements of any kind, as a precaution against their contraindicating (reacting adversely) with other treatments being administered.

Weight Gain and Difficulty Losing

This problem symptom may be one of the most concerning and is probably second only to unrelieved fatigue. Weight gain is a very frustrating symptom and one thyroid patients have strong desire to see corrected through their treatments.

This problem is more common in hypothyroid patients because hyperthyroidism typically causes weight loss rather than weight gain. Hyperthyroid patients however, do become hypothyroid if their case requires thyroid removal by surgical thyroidectomy or radioactive iodine ablation. It typically requires extra effort for treated hypothyroid patients to lose weight and to control it.

It is very important that hypothyroidism is adequately treated because under-treatment can contribute to weight problems from slowed metabolism and body fluid retention (myxedema). There are many diet plans available however; the keys to weight loss and control include the following.

• reducing calorie intake (i.e. simple carbohydrates: candies, pies, cookies and soft drinks)

• eating healthy foods (i.e. fruits, vegetables, nuts and grains)

• eliminating refined sugars as much as possible

• regular exercise

The claims of magical diets or ones that take no effort are usually false and weight loss remedies containing stimulants can be unhealthy and dangerous in some cases.

Joint and Muscle Aches

Many hypothyroid patients report that their first symptoms of thyroid disease were rheumatic ones, meaning joint and muscle aches and stiffness. Some patients in fact were believed to be experiencing Fibromyalgia Syndrome before receiving definitive diagnoses of thyroid disorders. Unfortunately some patients retain a degree of rheumatic symptoms even when well-treated. According the medical research studies, this can be due to "thyroid autoimmunity", meaning thyroid disease caused by auto-antibodies. These thyroid antibodies cause a degree of inflammation in the body which can settle in muscles and joints, causing mild to moderate aches and stiffness.

If rheumatic symptoms are severe and there is swelling or redness around joints, tests to detect or rule out Rheumatoid Arthritis (RA) should be conducted. Autoimmune thyroid diseases place patients at higher risk for other autoimmune conditions, including RA. When these type symptoms are thyroid-related, making sure replacement hormone therapy is at the proper level is important and some medical research has shown that supplementing with the mineral selenium may also help lower auto-antibody activity.

Over-the-counter anti-inflammatory drugs can also help reduce symptoms but these and any other drugs or supplements, should be approved by the patient's treating doctor, as a precaution against their interfering with other treatments currently being administered.

Emotional Symptoms

This area of symptomology is also common in both hypothyroid and hyperthyroid disorders as addressed in a previous chapter. Anxiety and/or depression can result from either type of thyroid hormone imbalance but medical research has also shown that emotional disorders can be associated with the disease process itself (thyroid autoimmunity). Most cases of hypothyroidism in industrialized countries are caused by "Hashimoto's thyroiditis" and most cases of hyperthyroidism are caused by Graves' disease. These are the autoimmune diseases that are the root cause. Medical research studies have concluded that the auto-antibodies that characterize these diseases may be responsible for emotional symptoms and disorders rather than abnormal hormone levels alone.

Patients with unresolved emotional disorder symptoms may need the added benefit of psychiatric therapies such as Cognitive Behavioral Therapy and/or psychotropic medications.

Prescription-medications that can help reduce anxiety and stress symptoms, include the following.

• benzodiazepines (i.e. Xanax)

• adrenergic receptor antagonists (i.e. Buspirone).

• daily regimen antidepressants - SSRI drugs (i.e. Paxil, Prozac, Zoloft)

Natural supplements that have been reported to help relieve anxiety and depression symptoms include the following.

• Bach's Rescue Remedy

• Panicyl

• St. John's Wort

• Valerian extract

• GABA

• SAMe

• Passion Flower

Any non-prescription supplements a patient may take need to be reported to their doctor to make sure he finds no risks of adverse reactions by adding them to medical treatments that are already being administered.

CHAPTER SIXTEEN

Treated Hypothyroidism and Fatigue

When Tiredness does Not Resolve with Thyroid Treatment

Feeling tired and fatigued is common in treated hypothyroid patients as addressed in a previous chapter. Surveys of treated patients have shown it to be one of the most common unresolved symptoms they experience. This chapter will be dedicated to further addressing this concerning and sometimes stubborn symptom.

When hypothyroid patients feel lack of energy or even totally exhausted despite being treated for hypothyroidism, there are several areas to consider, that might hold an answer to this lingering problem.

Optimized Thyroid Hormone Replacement

The first thing to consider when a patient continues to feel tired after being treated for hypothyroidism is whether or not their thyroid hormone therapy is at optimal or sub-optimal levels. Patients often have a narrow treatment range where the best symptom relief can be found or what might be referred to as their "set-point" as mentioned in an earlier chapter. This is that optimal level of thyroid hormone dose that best relieves their symptoms of hypothyroidism.

If for example, a patient has been treated to get their T4 and T3 thyroid hormone levels at approximately mid-range or only slightly above and their TSH level is still above lower-normal, this would suggest that a dose increase can be administered by the treating doctor in attempt toward better symptom-relief. This might be referred to as "wiggle room" to safely tweak the dose for better results.

TSH is suppressed with a thyroid hormone dose when it is elevated due to hypothyroidism. If for example, lowest normal at the blood lab used to monitor a hypothyroid patient's hormone therapy is "0.05" (a half-point) but their TSH has only been suppressed down to about 3.0 (three points), a trial of a dose to suppress it further down to about 1.0 should not place them at risk for over treatment (dose induced thyrotoxicity). If T4 and T3 levels stay within higher-normal range at this TSH level, this too would be reassurance against over-treatment and might also yield a much better level of symptom-relief for fatigue.

Thorough Blood Lab Evaluation

Hypothyroid patients are at higher risk for other problems, such as anemia, including the type caused by low vitamin B12 levels, celiac disease (intolerance to gluten in the diet), diabetes and problems with adrenal and sex hormone levels.

If fatigue or other symptoms continue in a hypothyroid patient who is well-treated and whose blood lab retests show that their thyroid hormone therapy dose has been optimized, thorough blood testing for these other disorders would be merited.

Each of these disorders can be detected or ruled out via diagnostic blood lab testing. In addition to complete blood counts, glucose levels, Vitamin B12, other hormone levels (i.e. sex and adrenal) and tests for antibodies that reveal Celiac disease (gluten-sensitive enteropathy), patients should also be tested for systemic autoimmunity via the ANA blood test and for systemic inflammation via the ESR blood test. These latter mentioned two tests can help to rule out or confirm other inflammatory and autoimmune diseases that may be present in the body, such as Lupus and Rheumatoid Arthritis, each of which can present with fatigue as a major symptom.

Thyroid Autoimmunity Contributes to Fatigue

While it is not often noted in medical studies or by doctors when communicating with their patients, "thyroid autoimmunity" (Hashimoto's thyroiditis) which is the most common cause of hypothyroidism in industrialized countries can also contribute to symptoms apart from corrected thyroid hormone levels.

Studies published on PubMed-U.S. National Institutes of Health - medical research website, state that thyroid autoimmunity (antibodies) can contribute to symptom manifestations ranging from rheumatic ones (joint and muscle problems) to severe life-threatening conditions such as Hashimoto's Ecephalopathy (rare inflammatory response in the brain). This can be true despite having abnormal thyroid hormone levels well-treated and corrected to optimal levels. Thyroid autoimmunity for example, is an inflammatory condition that can cause goiter as a first symptom, before thyroid hormone levels fall out of the normal range.

Supplements and Methods that can help Fatigue

When treatment for hypothyroidism has been optimized and other co-existing problems addressed or ruled out, additional steps can be taken to help with unrelieved fatigue. Natural supplements that can help energy levels include B vitamins, such as B-5, B-6 and B-12. There are sublingual brands of B-12 available (liquid for under the tongue) that can help maintain energy by dosing two to three times a day as needed. Many brands of B12 are formulated with Vitamin C added to help with absorption and are a combination that is helpful for healthy adrenal gland function as well.

Other natural supplements (not exceeded at manufacturer's recommended dose) that can help with fatigue include.

• coenzyme Q10

• folic acid

• thiamine

• niacin

• tyrosine

The effectiveness of some nutrients and vitamins do however also depend upon a healthy diet to work well in the body. It bears repeating that eliminating refined sugars and stimulants like caffeine and alcohol and eating plenty of fruits, vegetables, nuts and grains can be helpful. Limiting any intake of goitrogen foods (listed previously) that have a lowering effect on thyroid hormones can also help. These foods are more problem-some if not fully cooked or not eaten in small, infrequent servings. To also mention again - exercise in moderation often helps with energy levels but should only be done at tolerance-level or can otherwise exacerbate fatigue levels.

If fatigue is chronic and all other causes have been eliminated, a diagnosis of Chronic Fatigue Syndrome might result. Both CFS and Fibromyalgia have been found to affect thyroid patients more commonly than the general public.

CHAPTER SEVENTEEN

Qualities Needed in Hypothyroid Treating Doctors

What to Look for in Thyroid Specialists

The symptoms of hypothyroidism can be concerning and severe to a thyroid patient. This, points to the great importance in a qualified hypothyroid treatment specialist.

People needing treatment for hypothyroidism should seek doctors who are qualified in optimizing thyroid hormone therapy the best possible for each of their patients but who also monitor their patients for potential co-morbid conditions and treatment complications.

Palpation for Goiter and Thyroid Nodules

The vast majority of hypothyroid patients have the condition due to diseased thyroid glands. Thyroid specializing doctors should check their new patients for goiter (thyroid gland swelling) and for thyroid nodules (tumorous growths) by palpation. This means the doctor uses fingertips to feel for growths within the thyroid gland that might merit further investigation if found.

Most thyroid nodules are not suspicious for being malignant (cancerous) but if one is found that is of significant size or that is singular and of a solid-texture (solid, cold nodule) rather than among a group of nodules (multi-nodular), additional testing would likely be ordered for further evaluation. These would be precautionary measures, to rule out the possibility of thyroid cancer and the risk for obstructed breathing and/or swallowing if goiters or nodules of significant size are found or those that pose a danger of growing larger.

Diagnostic Blood Testing

Thyroid specializing doctors should not limit diagnosis of thyroid disorders to the TSH blood test only. He or she should also not limit the monitoring of thyroid hormone replacement therapy with the TSH level alone. Some thyroid hormone disorders may present with normal TSH levels such as certain types of secondary hypothyroidism. This includes cases of Central Hypothyroidism when TSH may test at normal values, low-normal or even below normal, with thyroid hormone levels (T4 and T3) also at below normal. TSH is supposed to elevate with hypothyroidism but fails to do so in these cases. The failure of TSH to rise can be due to a problem in the pituitary, the brain-gland that regulates thyroid function.

Thorough Monitoring of Newly-Treated Hypothyroid Patients

While TSH is accurate in monitoring thyroid hormone therapy in most cases, if central Hypothyroidism is being treated, the T4 and/or T3 thyroid hormones will also need to be tested. It is also a reasonable precaution to test thyroid hormone levels in addition to TSH in all newly-treated hypothyroid patients for at least the first couple of follow-up blood retests, to make sure both T4 and T3 are staying at proper levels and are correlating properly with TSH. Once it is determined that TSH is all that is needed to monitor a patient's treatment, the doctor can at that time switch to using it as the only test.

Newly treated hypothyroid patients should be blood retested at no longer than 3-month intervals, while patients who are stable on a dose of replacement thyroid hormone that has reached optimal level, may only need retested once every 6-months. A treating doctor should also instruct their patients to report any symptoms that may appear between blood retests that might indicate either over-treatment (hyperthyroid) or under-treatment (hypothyroid) and the possible need for a dose adjustment.

Adjusting Thyroid Hormone Replacement Doses

Some thyroid doctors have targeted treatment goals rather than simply treating hypothyroid patients on replacement hormone doses to get their levels anywhere within normal values. However, less than mid-range normal values for the T4 and T3 or low-normal values may keep some patients in a state of unrelieved hypothyroid symptoms.

Doctors who are more targeted to achieve best results for their hypothyroid patients will be willing to adjust their doses of hormone therapy to reach at least mid-range or higher-normal T4 and T3 levels. This may require suppressing the TSH to very low-normal readings in some patients and will require that the treating doctor is willing to make the needed dose adjustments to reach the target therapy goal.

Some patients may see more symptom relief with a different type of prescription thyroid hormone (T4 only or combination T4/T3) or a different brand (synthetic or natural) and a doctor should be willing to switch patients to a trial of another type if the initial brand they started treatment with yields unsatisfactory results.

(END)